Neuroendovascular Management: Cranial/Spinal Disorders

Guest Editors

ROBERT H. ROSENWASSER, MD, FACS, FAHA
PASCAL M. JABBOUR, MD

NEUROSURGERY CLINICS OF NORTH AMERICA

www.neurosurgery.theclinics.com

Consulting Editors
ANDREW T. PARSA, MD, PhD
PAUL C. McCORMICK, MD, MPH

October 2009 • Volume 20 • Number 4

SAUNDERS an imprint of ELSEVIER, Inc.

W.B. SAUNDERS COMPANY
A Division of Elsevier Inc.

1600 John F. Kennedy Blvd. • Suite 1800 • Philadelphia, PA 19103-2899

http://www.theclinics.com

NEUROSURGERY CLINICS OF NORTH AMERICA Volume 20, Number 4
October 2009 ISSN 1042-3680, ISBN-13: 978-1-4377-1574-3, ISBN-10: 1-4377-1574-5

Editor: Ruth Malwitz
Developmental Editor: Donald Mumford

Neurosurgery Clinics of North America (ISSN 1042-3680) is published quarterly by Elsevier Inc., 360 Park Avenue South, New York, NY 10010-1710. Months of issue are January, April, July, and October. Business and Editorial Offices: 1600 John F. Kennedy Blvd., Suite 1800, Philadelphia, PA 19103-2899. Customer Service Office: 11830 Westline Industrial Drive, St. Louis, MO 63146. Periodicals postage paid at New York, NY, and additional mailing offices. Subscription prices are $274.00 per year (US individuals), $438.00 per year (US institutions), $300.00 per year (Canadian individuals), $535.00 per year (Canadian institutions), $383.00 per year (international individuals), $535.00 per year (international institutions), $138.00 per year (US students), and $189.00 per year (international students). International air speed delivery is included in all *Clinics* subscription prices. All prices are subject to change without notice. **POSTMASTER:** Send address changes to *Neurosurgery Clinics of North America*, Elsevier Periodicals Customer Service, 11830 Westline Industrial Drive, St. Louis, MO 63146. **Customer Service: 1-800-654-2452 (US and Canada). From outside the US and Canada, call: 1-314-453-7041. Fax: 1-314-453-5170. E-mail:** JournalsCustomerService-usa@elsevier.com **(for print support) and** journalsonlinesupport-usa@elsevier.com **(for online support).**

Reprints. For copies of 100 or more, of articles in this publication, please contact the Commercial Reprints Department, Elsevier Inc., 360 Park Avenue South, New York, NY 10010-1710. Tel. (212) 633-3812; Fax: (212) 462-1935; E-mail: reprints@elsevier.com.

Neurosurgery Clinics of North America is covered in *MEDLINE/PubMed (Index Medicus), EMBASE/Excerpta Medica, and Current Contents/Clinical Medicine (CC/CM).*

Printed and bound by CPI Group (UK) Ltd, Croydon, CR0 4YY

Transferred to Digital Print 2011

Contributors

GUEST EDITORS

ROBERT H. ROSENWASSER, MD, FACS, FAHA
Professor and Chairman, Department of Neurological Surgery; Professor, Department of Radiology; Professor, Division of Cerebrovascular Surgery and Interventional Neuroradiology, Thomas Jefferson University, Jefferson Hospital for Neuroscience, Philadelphia, Pennsylvania

PASCAL M. JABBOUR, MD
Assistant Professor, Department of Neurological Surgery, Thomas Jefferson University, Jefferson Hospital for Neuroscience, Philadelphia, Pennsylvania

AUTHORS

JASON ALLEN, MD
Department of Radiology, New York University Langone Medical Center, New York, New York

TIBOR BESCKE, MD
Assistant Professor, Department of Neurology, New York University Langone Medical Center, New York, New York

ARUNDHATI BISWAS, MD
Department of Neurosurgery, Harborview Medical Center, University of Washington, Seattle, Washington

JAMES DOUGLAS, MD
Department of Radiation Oncology, Harborview Medical Center, University of Washington, Seattle, Washington

BASAVARAJ GHODKE, MD
Department of Neurosurgery, Harborview Medical Center, University of Washington, Seattle, Washington

DANIAL HALLAM, MD
Departments of Neurosurgery and Radiology, Harborview Medical Center, University of Washington, Seattle, Washington

PASCAL M. JABBOUR, MD
Assistant Professor, Department of Neurological Surgery, Thomas Jefferson University, Jefferson Hospital for Neuroscience, Philadelphia, Pennsylvania

MICHELE H. JOHNSON, MD
Associate Professor, Departments of Diagnostic Radiology, Surgery (Otolaryngology), and Neurosurgery; Director of Interventional Neuroradiology, Yale University School of Medicine, New Haven, Connecticut

LOUIS J. KIM, MD
Department of Neurosurgery and Department of Radiology, Harborview Medical Center, University of Washington, Seattle, Washington

SEAN D. LAVINE, MD
Director of Endovascular Neurosurgery, Department of Neurosurgery and Radiology, Columbia University, College of Physicians and Surgeons, New York, New York

KATHLEEN A. McCONNELL, MD
Resident, Department of Radiology, New York University Langone Medical Center, New York

PETER K. NELSON, MD
Associate Professor, Departments of
Radiology and Neurosurgery, New York
University Langone Medical Center, New York,
New York

RAUL G. NOGUEIRA, MD
Department of Neurology, Massachusetts
General Hospital/Harvard Medical School,
Boston, Massachusetts

**ROBERT H. ROSENWASSER, MD,
FACS, FAHA**
Professor and Chairman, Department of
Neurological Surgery; Professor, Department
of Radiology; Professor, Division of
Cerebrovascular Surgery and Interventional
Neuroradiology, Thomas Jefferson University,
Jefferson Hospital for Neuroscience,
Philadelphia, Pennsylvania

LALIGAM N. SEKHAR, MD, FACS
Departments of Neurosurgery, Radiology, and
Neurological Surgery, Harborview Medical
Center, Seattle, Washington

MAKSIM SHAPIRO, MD
Department of Radiology, New York University
Langone Medical Center, New York,
New York

DOROTHEA STROZYK, MD
Departments of Neurosurgery and Radiology,
Columbia University College of Physicians and
Surgeons, New York, New York

HJALTI M. THORISSON, MD
Attending Radiologist, Department of
Radiology, University Hospital of Iceland,
Reykjavik, Iceland; Adjunct Assistant Professor,
Department of Diagnostic Radiology, Yale
University School of Medicine, New Haven,
Connecticut

STAVROPOULA I. TJOUMAKARIS, MD
Instructor, Department of Neurosurgery,
Thomas Jefferson University, Jefferson
Hospital for Neuroscience, Philadelphia,
Pennsylvania

Contents

classification, symptomatology, and treatment. Endovascular therapy is rapidly progressing to an adjunct or even alternative treatment to microsurgical resection. Several techniques, such as transarterial or transvenous embolization with metallic coils, NBCA, or Onyx, have been used successfully in several studies. The long-term clinical and radiographic outcomes of endovascular therapy for the treatment of dural arteriovenous fistulas are satisfactory, and future studies are underway for the refinement of these techniques.

Cerebral vasospasm continues to be the leading treatable cause of death and disability in patients with subarachnoid hemorrhage. Transluminal balloon angioplasty has been considered a safe and effective treatment for cerebral vasospasm resistant to maximal medical treatment. However, it should be performed in a timely manner, any delays could potentially increase the risk of hemorrhagic infarct. Angioplasty in the affected territory may be of benefit in improving not only the angiographic appearance but also the ultimate outcome for the patient, if performed in a timely fashion.

Carotid-cavernous fistulae are abnormal arterial communications within the cavernous sinus. Endovascular obliteration is the mainstay therapy for the definitive treatment of these lesions. Several approaches have been described. These include transarterial or transvenous embolization with balloons, coils, particles, or covered stents, and arterial sacrifice. The preferred technique is based on the fistula type (direct or indirect), microanatomy, chronicity, and the extent of the arterial defect.

Endovascular procedures are rapidly expanding as treatment options for cerebrovascular diseases and neoplasms of the head and neck and are becoming less invasive but more effective. There are potentially dangerous anastomoses between the extracranial and intracranial circulations; hence, thorough knowledge of the anatomy is essential to minimize the risk of cranial nerve palsies, blindness, or neurologic deficits. It is essential to understand the scientific basis of treatment rationale based on advancing new neuroimaging techniques to better serve patients. An interdisciplinary approach and treatment in high-volume centers are vital to obtain maximal benefit for patients.

Endovascular therapies have become a mainstream option for treatment of many extracranial vascular disorders and is the preferred management strategy for vascular injury secondary to head and neck malignancy. The interventionalist must be familiar with the clinical trials as basis for the management of extracranial athero-sclerotic disease as well as understanding the therapeutic options, risks, and benefits. Nonatherosclerotic injury including trauma, injury due to neoplasm or its treatment, and idiopathic lesions have unique considerations important to the use and deployment of various devices. The diagnostic approaches, treatment strategies, and the role of endovascular techniques in patients with extracranial vascular disease are discussed.

Neurosurgery Clinics of North America

THE CLINICS ARE NOW AVAILABLE ONLINE!

Access your subscription at:
www.theclinics.com

Preface

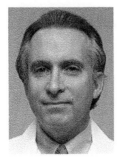
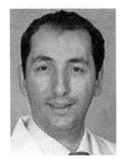

Robert H. Rosenwasser, MD,   Pascal M. Jabbour, MD
FACS, FAHA

Guest Editors

This is the second of 2 issues in a series on current thoughts, concepts, and the practice of neuroendovascular therapy. It deals with different neurovascular pathologies and their endovascular treatment, visiting different subjects from tumor embolizations to carotid cavernous fistulae, intracranial aneurysms, vasospasm, arteriovenous malformations, stroke, carotid and vertebral disease, and dural arteriovenous malformation.

The authors of this issue come from backgrounds in neurology, neurosurgery, and interventional neuroradiology, demonstrating the way in which the various disciplines have come together for better patient care. They are leaders in the field and have contributed a great deal. We wish to acknowledge all of the authors for their diligence and effort in preparing their contributions for this issue.

We feel certain that you will find this issue timely and informative. It will undoubtedly be the mainstay of references for some time to come.

Robert H. Rosenwasser, MD, FACS, FAHA
Pascal M. Jabbour, MD

Department of Neurological Surgery
Thomas Jefferson University
Jefferson Hospital for Neuroscience
909 Walnut Street, 3rd floor
Philadelphia, PA 19107, USA

E-mail address:
robert.rosenwasser@jefferson.edu
(R.H. Rosenwasser)

Neurosurg Clin N Am 20 (2009) ix
doi:10.1016/j.nec.2009.07.016
1042-3680/09/$ – see front matter © 2009 Elsevier Inc. All rights reserved.

neurosurgery.theclinics.com

Endovascular Management of Intracranial Aneurysms

Pascal M. Jabbour, MD*, Stavropoula I. Tjoumakaris, MD,
Robert H. Rosenwasser, MD, FACS, FAHA

KEYWORDS

• Aneurysm • Endovascular • Coil • Stent • Embolization

Cerebral aneurysms are thought to arise from weakness within the tunica media of the vessel thus allowing for expansion of the vascular wall with time and introduction of inciting factors such as smoking and hypertension. Cerebral aneurysms form at regions where there is stress related to turbulent flow. Such stress is most commonly present at branching points within the Circle of Willis. Greater than 80% of aneurysms are present within the anterior circulation while 10% to 20% arise within the posterior circulation.

Risk factors that increase the probability of developing cerebral aneurysms are polycystic kidney disease, aortic coarctation, alpha-1antitrypsin deficiency, Ehler's-Danlos Type IV, fibromuscular dysplasia, and a family history of cerebral aneurysms.[1–3] Patients harboring cerebral aneurysms are usually diagnosed because of symptoms related to rupture and thus development of subarachnoid hemorrhage (SAH), or mass effect on cerebral structures as the aneurysm expands, or cerebral ischemia from thrombus formation within the aneurismal sac. Nonetheless, screening has led to the diagnosis of asymptomatic patients. There is a four times higher incidence of aneurysms within first-degree relatives of patients presenting with subarachnoid hemorrhage.[4]

The International Study of Unruptured Intracranial Aneurysms (ISUIA) has defined the natural history of asymptomatic intracranial aneurysms.[5] The 5-year rupture rate based on size is as follows for anterior circulation aneurysms not including posterior communicating artery aneurysms (PCom): 0% for less than 7 mm, 2.6% for 7 to 12 mm, 14.5% for 13 to 24 mm, and 40% for greater than 25 mm. The same rates for PCom and posterior circulation aneurysms is as follows: 2.5% for less than 7 mm, 14.5% for 7 to 12 mm, 18.4% for 13 to 24 mm, and 50% for greater than 25 mm.[5]

The consensus has been that individuals 60 years of age or younger harboring intracranial aneurysm of equal to or greater than 7 mm should be offered treatment. Within our own practice, most patients presenting with SAH harbor aneurysms smaller than 10 mm and some even smaller than 5 mm. Individuals who have severe headaches, family history of SAH, or use tobacco are at a higher risk of rupture and thus are offered treatment of aneurysms at less than 7 mm.

Patients who present with SAH have a 15% immediate mortality and a 50% mortality at 6 months.[6,7] Clinical outcome is related to the presenting clinical condition of the patient.[8] Such an outcome is related to rerupture of the aneurysm as well as delayed neurologic deficits related to spasm of the intracranial vasculature.[9–11] Treatment of the ruptured aneurysm and the related vasospasm and hydrocephalus has led to better outcomes.

The endovascular treatment of cerebral aneurysms has seen an exponential growth since the Food and Drug Administration (FDA) approval of Guglielmi detachable coils (GDCs) in 1995. Advances in interventional neuroradiology led to

Department of Neurological Surgery, Thomas Jefferson University Hospital, Jefferson Hospital for Neuroscience, 909 Walnut Street, 3rd Floor, Philadelphia, PA 19107, USA
* Corresponding author.
E-mail address: pascal.jabbour@jefferson.edu (P.M. Jabbour).

Neurosurg Clin N Am 20 (2009) 383–398
doi:10.1016/j.nec.2009.07.003
1042-3680/09/$ – see front matter © 2009 Elsevier Inc. All rights reserved.

significant improvement in catheter and guide wire technology and digital angiography equipment is evolving continuously. As a result, the use of endovascular techniques in the management of cerebral aneurysms has progressed from an alternative to surgery for inaccessible lesions to a frontline treatment. Indeed, the International Subarachnoid Aneursym Trial (ISAT) showed a favorable outcome in patients undergoing endovascular aneurysm occlusion compared with clipping ligation in the ruptured patient population.[12] Radiographic and clinical follow-up is essential for the determination of aneurysm occlusion and future hemorrhage risks.

PATIENT SELECTION

Careful consideration of the patient's clinical presentation and aneurysm characteristics contributes to the decision to occlude a cerebral aneurysm using an endovascular approach.[13]

The age of the patient in combination with other medical comorbidities plays a significant role in decision making. Patients of advanced age are less likely to withstand extensive intracranial surgery and more likely to be considered for the endovascular approach. Although the decision to manage cerebral aneurysms in the elderly remains extremely difficult, several studies in patients older than 70 years of age have proven that endovascular embolization is both safe and effective.[14,15]

Medical comorbidities should be thoroughly assessed before aneurysm occlusion. Patients with a complex medical history, in particular poorly controlled diabetes, severe cardiac disease, chronic obstructive pulmonary disease, bleeding diathesis, and thrombotic disease requiring chronic anticoagulation, are generally considered for endovascular management. Implementation of perioperative medical management by appropriate consulting teams is important to minimize patient risks and complications.

In the SAH patient population, clinical grade on presentation is also important. Patients with poor clinical grade (Hunt and Hess grade IV or V) are potential candidates for endovascular aneurysm treatment. In our institution, Hunt and Hess grade V patients are generally considered for endovascular management following clinical improvement with placement of ventriculostomy.

Ideally, aneurysms with a narrow inflow region (neck) and therefore a large fundus to neck ratio have better endovascular outcomes. As a rule, giant and fusiform aneurysms are not good candidates for endovascular treatment. Aneurysm location could also affect treatment options. Middle cerebral artery (MCA) aneurysms present with

technical difficulties for endovascular occlusion and should first be considered for microsurgical clipping. In contrast, posterior circulation aneurysms, especially with brainstem projection or complex morphology, are better treated via the endovascular approach.[16] Other possible candidates for this approach are patients with multiple aneurysms and an unknown source of rupture, as well as patients with sidewall aneurysms.

Finally, the cerebrovascular patient anatomy could influence the choice of the treatment modality. The presence of significant vasospasm, turtuosity of proximal vessels, moderate atherosclerosis, and very distally located aneurysms is usually contraindicated for endovascular techniques.

TECHNICAL ASPECT

All endovascular procedures should be performed under general endotracheal anesthesia and continuous somatosensory evoked potential and electroencephalography recordings. An appropriate choice of anesthetic agent is required to maintain intraoperative anesthesia and prevent increases in intracranial and cardiovascular pressures. In posterior circulation and PCom artery aneurysms, brainstem auditory evoked potentials are also monitored.[17] For ruptured aneurysms, intracranial pressure monitoring with a ventriculostomy and hemodynamic monitoring with a Swan-Ganz catheter are highly recommended in patients with Hunt and Hess grades of III and above.

Anticoagulation with continuous heparin infusion is routinely used in all embolization procedures. The use of activated clotting time (ACT) is recommended for close monitoring of systemic anticoagulation. A baseline ACT value is obtained for each patient before heparinization. Satisfactory anticoagulation is achieved when the new ACT value has increased by 2.0 to 2.5 from the baseline.[17] In addition, intraluminar air is carefully avoided with frequent system checks before and during the procedure.

Arterial access is obtained through femoral puncture and an arterial sheath is inserted and secured with a stitch. Arterial navigation through the aorta to the carotid artery is performed with a guiding catheter. Radiopaque markings on all guiding catheters and wires are instrumental for successful navigation and coil delivery. When the aneurysm location is unknown, a six-vessel angiogram is recommended, including bilateral external carotid, internal carotid, and vertebral arteries. Digital cerebral angiography is used to determine the optimal skull angle for treatment. In some cases, a three-dimensional (3-D) vascular reconstruction allows for thorough visualization of complex or small aneurysms. A microcatheter is then inserted in the parent vessel and navigated toward the aneurysm via a road map technique. A road map is obtained by intra-arterial contrast injection followed by digital subtraction of sequential images. A microguide wire within the microcatheter is used for steering and for introduction of the microcatheter into the aneurysm lumen by placement of the former into the inflow zone. Careful withdrawal of the wire and advancement of the microcatheter into the aneurysm is then performed.[16]

Endovascular aneurysm obliteration could be broadly classified into two approaches: the reconstructive approach focuses on selective aneurysm occlusion, whereas the deconstructive approach achieves aneurysm obliteration by parent vessel occlusion. The choice of the appropriate method depends on multiple factors such as aneurysm location, size, shape, and presence of collateral cerebral blood flow.

THE JEFFERSON HOSPITAL FOR NEUROSCIENCE EXPERIENCE
Patient Selection

From July 1994 through December 2004, 2721 patients were treated for intracranial aneurysms at Thomas Jefferson University Hospital and Jefferson Hospital for Neuroscience.[17] The age range was 9 to 89 years involving a cohort of 72% women and 18% of patients with multiple aneurysms. The clinical presentation upon treatment included 599 (22%) patients with unruptured aneurysms and 2122 (78%) patients with acute subarachnoid hemorrhage. Most patients treated were either Grade III or Grade IV. Hunt-Hess grade was as follows: 8% Grade I, 20% Grade II, 62% Grade III, 10% Grade IV (**Box 1**). No patients who remained a Grade V after ventricular drainage and aggressive critical care support underwent diagnostic angiography.

Our cohort of patients with intracranial aneurysms underwent transcranial surgery in 1414 patients (52%) and endovascular treatment in 1307 patients (48%). Aneurysm location for endovascular treatment involved 66% anterior circulation and 34% posterior circulation. **Box 2** outlines our criteria for selecting coil embolization versus craniotomy for clip ligation. The patients were individualized based on physiologic age and surgical, medical, and anesthetic risk factors using American Society of Anesthesiology classification and Goldman classification for cardiovascular risk factors as well as neurologic grade (**Fig. 1**). In general, poor neurologic-grade patients,

regardless of age, were selected to undergo an endovascular procedure. The presence of a large intraparenchymal hematoma, regardless of the aforementioned, would undergo transcranial surgery for relief of intracranial pressure and treatment of the aneurysm at the same time. More recently several patients underwent a combined treatment of endosaccular aneurysm occlusion followed by immediate surgery for transcranial removal of the hematoma. Small hematomas either in the temporal lobe or frontal lobe were not contraindications to endosaccular treatment and heparinization. Difficult or high-risk anatomic locations, such as posterior circulation aneurysms including low-lying or posteriorly pointing basilar aneurysms, were selected for an endovascular approach as well (**Fig. 2**). Endovascular treatment was usually excluded for giant aneurysms, aneurysms with thrombus, fusiform lesions, and unfavorable aneurysm fundus-to-neck ratio. Indications have expanded with balloon remodeling techniques and more recently with the Neuroform stent-assisted coiling procedure. Newer complex

---

Box 1
Hunt-Hess grade for 2122 SAH patients treated at Jefferson Hospital for Neuroscience between July 1994 and December 2004

- Grade 1: 169 patients (8%)
- Grade 2: 425 patients (20%)
- Grade 3: 1316 patients (62%)
- Grade 4: 212 patients (10%)
- Grade 5: Not treated if remained GR 5 after ventricular drainage, aggressive critical care support.

Box 2
Selection criteria for endovascular treatment

Inclusion factors:

- Elderly - "physiologic age"
- High surgical risk - medical and anesthetic risk
- Poor neurologic grade
- No intraparenchymal hematoma-"negotiable"
- Difficult/high risk - anatomic location-proximal ICA, posterior circulation
- Inability to surgically occlude

Relative exclusion factors (no longer absolute with stent/balloon-assist techniques):

- Giant aneurysm with/without thrombus
- Fusiform lesion
- Unfavorable fundus/neck ratio

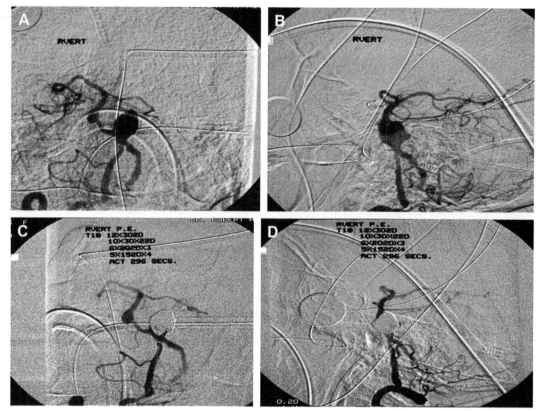

Fig. 1. An ideal endovascular candidate. (*A, B*) Oblique anteroposterior (AP) and lateral views demonstrating an unruptured vertebro-basilar junction aneurysm with a favorable fundus-neck ratio in an 87-year-old woman with heart failure and ejection fraction of 20%. (*C, D*) Postembolization views demonstrating complete obliteration.

coils that retain shape have allowed safer treatment of aneurysms with unfavorable morphology. Giant aneurysms and those with thrombus remain difficult to treat endovascularly because of a high recurrence rate and increased thromboembolic risk. Coil embolization has been a useful multimodality component combined with surgical clipping and/or vessel deconstruction for these lesions. **Figs. 3–8** illustrate the evolution in treatment modality selection over the past 5 years as new coil technologies have allowed a greater percentage of aneurysms to be successfully treated by endovascular means.

Clinical Results

We have recently reviewed our outcomes with endovascular management of posterior circulation aneurysms. The breakdown of aneurysm location involved 60% basilar apex, 20% posterior inferior cerebellar artery, 12% posterior communicating artery, 5% superior cerebellar artery, 4% anterior inferior cerebellar artery with 8 technical failures treated with microsurgery. Angiographic outcomes were 80% complete obliteration and 20% partial neck remnant. Clinical outcomes based on Glasgow Outcome Scores were 90.0% excellent or good, 5.0% fair, 2.5% poor, and 2.5% mortality. Procedural complications occurred in 6% of cases, mostly involving transient morbidity from thromboembolic events. We have also analyzed outcomes of coil embolization of 46 ruptured MCA aneurysms resulting in an independent outcome (mRs 0–2) for 85% of Hunt and Hess 1-3 patients and a complete or near complete obliteration rate of 93% for all patients. Our overall experience has demonstrated both a learning curve and growth of technology reducing the technical failure rate of 16% noted within the first 6 years to 8% for the past 5 years. To date, 7.2% of patients have required retreatment because of recurrence; longer follow-up is demonstrating that this number is increasing. Beginning in December 2003, Neuroform stent-assisted coiling was used for patients who could not be treated without this technique because of a fundus-to-neck ratio of less than 2. There were a total of 172 patients with 165 deployments. Initial angiographic outcomes showed a complete occlusion rate of 95%. Initially, with the first-generation

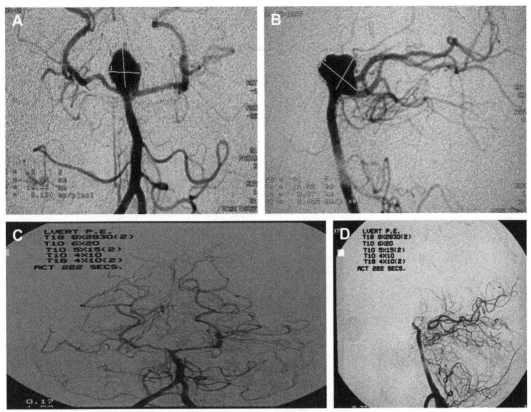

Fig. 2. Role of anatomic location and neurologic grade in treatment selection. (*A, B*) AP and lateral views demonstrating posteriorly pointing basilar apex aneurysm in a 38-year-old man HH 3 SAH. (*C, D*) Postembolization views demonstrating complete obliteration.

delivery system, there were seven failures to deploy. All patients had attempted coil embolization without stent placement. There were two strokes, primarily related to stent placement within the M1 segment with perforator and lenticulostriate occlusion. We have had five patients experience transient ischemic attacks (TIAs) with no angiographic etiology. There has been a higher complication rate with stent-assisted coil embolization for MCA aneurysms and for recurrent aneurysms previously embolized.

CLINICAL TRIAL OUTCOMES

One of the earliest prospective studies published on GDC aneurysm treatment involved 403 patients treated at eight centers in an FDA trial leading to approval in 1995.[18] Patients were selected for coil embolization owing to "surgical exclusion" risk factors including difficult size or location in 69%, failed surgical exploration in 13%, poor neurologic status in 12%, and poor medical status in 5%. Aneurysm dome morphology was 61% small (4–10 mm), 35% large (10–24 mm), 4% giant with neck size small (<4 mm) in 54%, wide in 36%, and fusiform in 6%. Aneurysm location was 57% posterior circulation with the three most common sites involving basilar bifurcation (31%), anterior communicating (13%), and posterior communicating (13%). Angiographic outcomes were dependent on aneurysm morphology with 71% complete occlusion rate in small aneurysms with a small neck versus 31% complete occlusion in small aneurysm with a wide neck. The overall morbidity and mortality rates were 8.9% and 6.2% respectively with intraprocedural rupture in 2.7%, thromboembolic events in 2.5%, and unintentional parent vessel occlusion in 3.0% with a rebleed rate of 2.2%. Although this preliminary data led to FDA approval, the long-term efficacy remained unknown.

Murayama and colleagues[19] provided a more recent review of an 11-year experience with 916 aneurysms at a single institution. They divided treatment groups into an early cohort treated from 1990 to 1995 and a latter cohort from 1995 to 2002. The overall rate of complete occlusion improved from 50% to 57% with fewer partial or

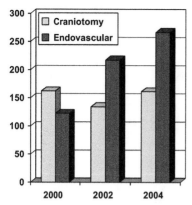

Fig. 3. Evolving practice paradigm toward endovascular treatment.

incomplete treatments in the latter group. The recanalization rate was 21% with a reduction from 26% to 17% between the initial and more recent groups. The technical complication rate

was 8.4%, comprised mostly of thromboembolic events and intraprocedural rupture. The overall rate of delayed aneurysm rupture was 1.6% but only 0.5% in the more recently treated cohort, predominately involving large or giant aneurysms. This study demonstrated better results with the evolution of newer coil techniques and technology; however, recanalization and rate of delayed rebleeding remained a concern requiring close follow-up imaging studies. Byrne and colleagues[20] reviewed a 5-year experience in England with 313 patients embolized after subarachnoid hemorrhage. They achieved complete occlusion in 64%, small remnant in 34%, and incomplete treatment in 2%. Follow-up angiography at 6 to 12 months postembolization demonstrated a stable occlusion in 85% and recurrence in 15% while there was progressive thrombosis in 8.5% of cases. Annual rebleeding rates were 0.8% in the first year, 0.6% in the second year, and 2.4% in the third year with no rebleeds in those followed

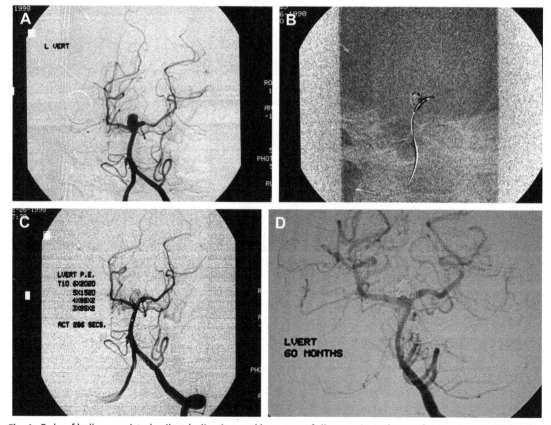

Fig. 4. Role of balloon-assisted coil embolization and long-term follow-up in endovascular treatment. (*A*) AP view of wide-necked basilar-P1 junction aneurysm in a 49-year-old patient HH4 SAH. (*B*) Intraoperative view of inflated balloon maintaining the microcatheter and coils within aneurysm neck during embolization. (*C*) Immediate postembolization view while fully anticoagulated showing small residual neck filling that was completely obliterated at 6-month follow-up. (*D*) The 60-month follow-up view showing complete obliteration despite a suggestion of recurrence on MRA.

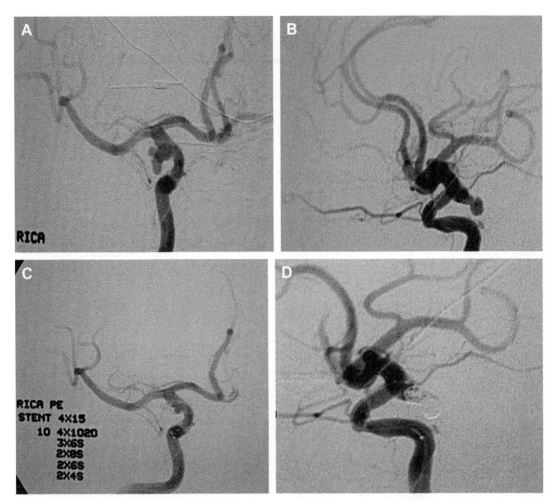

Fig. 5. Angiograms of a 54-year-old woman with Hunt and Hess grade IV subarachnoid hemorrhage from a ruptured right PCom artery aneurysm. (*A, B*) AP and lateral views of right ICA injection. The patient was treated with stent-assisted coiling. (*C, D*) AP and lateral views of right ICA injection following treatment.

beyond 3 years. Rebleeding occurred in 3 (7.9%) of 38 aneurysms with an unstable occlusion and 1 (0.4%) of 221 aneurysms with a stable occlusion observed on 6-month follow-up angiography. Raymond and colleagues[21] demonstrated that recurrent aneurysms have a low incidence of re-bleeding in a retrospective review of 501 aneurysms with a recurrence rate of 33.6% over 12 months average angiographic follow-up but a hemorrhage rate of only 0.8% over a mean clinical follow-up of 31 months.

The success documented in several retrospective and prospective series on endovascular treatment led to a need for level I evidence.[22–24] Koivisto and colleagues[25] provided a small prospective randomized trial comparing endovascular and surgical clipping outcomes of ruptured aneurysms in 109 patients. They found no difference in Glasgow Outcome Scores and neuropsychological testing at 12 months post treatment between the two groups. Angiographic obliteration rates were better in the surgical clipping arm (86% vs 77% complete) with no delayed re-hemorrhages at 1 year in either group. The most comprehensive study to date is the ISAT trial.[12] This study identified 9559 patients with ruptured aneurysms and randomized the 2143 patients deemed by both the open surgical and endovascular teams to be amenable to either treatment. The primary outcome assessment was a modified Rankin score of 3 to 6 (dependent or dead) at 1 year clinical follow-up. The study concluded the endovascular group had a relative and absolute risk reduction in disability or death of 22.6% and 6.9%, respectively, which was significantly better than the surgical group. The

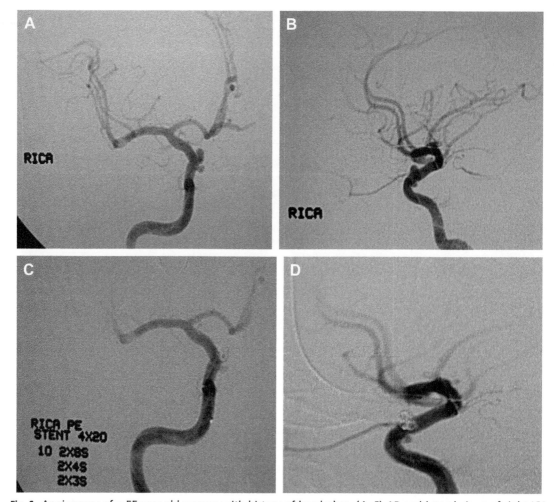

Fig. 6. Angiograms of a 55-year-old woman with history of headaches. (*A, B*) AP and lateral views of right ICA injection. A right-sided wide-neck paraclinoid aneurysm and cavernous aneurysm are noted. The patient was treated with stent-assisted coiling of the paraclinoid aneurysm. (*C, D*) AP and lateral views of right ICA injection following treatment.

study also found a low cumulative rebleeding rate in both treatment groups, although slightly more frequent in the endovascular group (0.15% vs 0.07%). Given the impact of this study particularly in the United States, critics were quick to question the outcomes of the more than 7000 patients not randomized, the potentially unequal level of experience for open surgical sites involved, the applicability beyond good grade patients (World Federation of Neurological Surgeons grade 1–3, 88%) and certain aneurysm morphology and location (size <10 mm, 93%; anterior circulation, 97%), and the lack of significant outcome difference in all mRs groups other than 3 to 6.[26] Clearly many questions surround this study but it remains the only level I evidence comparing endovascular to open surgical treatment of ruptured aneurysms.

RECONSTRUCTIVE APPROACH
Guglielmi Detachable Coil System

Guglielmi detachable coils (GDCs) are made of a soft platinum alloy attached to a stainless steel deliver wire.[27] Coils of varying softness, size, helical diameter, and length are currently available. Newer generation coils have a 3-D shape, coating materials, and complex helical patterns, allowing for precise obliteration of the aneurysm sac.

Once the microcatheter is inserted into the aneurysm lumen, the platinum coils are introduced under direct angiographic guidance. The mean arterial pressure should be carefully lowered by 15% to 20% during coil deployment, particularly in the acute hemorrhagic cases.[17] The initial coil is carefully chosen by its ability to bridge the aneurysm neck and facilitate dense and

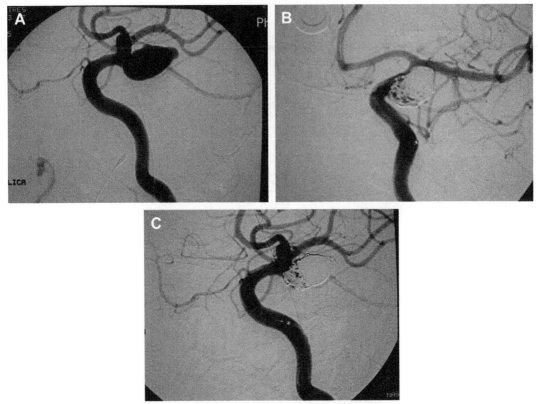

Fig. 7. Angiograms of a 62-year-old male with Hunt and Hess grade III subarachnoid hemorrhage. (*A*) Lateral view of left ICA injection showing a giant PCom artery aneurysm. The patient was treated with endovascular coiling embolization. (*B, C*) AP and lateral views of left ICA injection following treatment.

homogeneous packing of the lumen. The first coil is usually the longest and is placed with a basketlike configuration. Multiple coils of similar or variable morphologies may be used for the embolization of each aneurysm. Coil detachment is performed electrically with delivery of a low-voltage current, once optimal coil positioning is achieved. The procedure is completed when aneurysm occlusion is maximized or surgeon discretion discourages further packing for fear of aneurysm rupture or parent vessel occlusion. The goal of endovascular treatment is lack of aneurysm filling under normotension and full anticoagulation, observed in multiple rotational views (at least 6).[17]

Stent-assisted Coiling Technique

The introduction of intravascular stents has expanded the therapeutic applications of coiling embolization to include complex or wide-neck aneurysms.[28] Similar to deployment of a coil through a microcatheter, a stent is placed across the aneurysm neck and detached with delivery of low-voltage current. The stent provides an endoluminal scaffold that prevents coil herniation into the parent vessel. Coil delivery into the aneurysm is achieved through the scaffold mesh into the lumen. The stent placement across the aneurysm neck could have an additional benefit in aneurysm obliteration by diverting cerebral blood flow away from the lumen and enhancing aneurysm thrombosis. Concerns with intra-arterial thrombus and embolus formation are addressed with long-term anticoagulation or antiplatelet therapies.

We had published our early results in stent-assisted coiling with a first-generation Neuroform stent[28] showing that it is a useful technique to treat wide-neck aneurysms, it still has its limitations, and the thromboembolic events remain a major concern.

Balloon-assisted Coiling Technique

Bilateral femoral access is obtained with a 7-French vascular sheath or use of a "Y" adapter using an 8-French sheath. A diagnostic angiography run is performed to try to select the best view of the neck and the branching vessels for the coiling procedure, with if needed a 3-D angiographic acquisition. After measurement of the

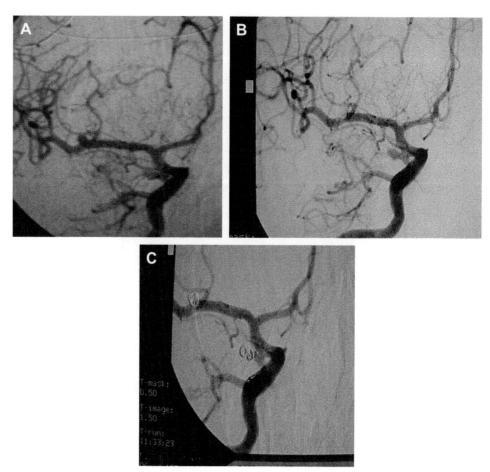

Fig. 8. Angiograms of a 43-year-old female with Hunt and Hess grade III subarachnoid hemorrhage. (*A*) AP view of right ICA injection showing an MCA and PCom aneurysms. The patient underwent coiling embolization of both aneurysms. (*B*) AP view of right ICA injection following treatment of MCA aneurysm. (*C*) AP view of right ICA injection following treatment of both aneurysms. Note the filling of PCom artery following embolization.

activated clotting time, a bolus of heparin is given with a goal to have the activated clotting time twice the baseline. Heparin may be maintained for 24 hours after the procedure but is generally decided by case-specific circumstances. The parent vessel is catheterized with a microcatheter that will be placed near the aneurysm neck. A nondetachable silicone balloon is then advanced through the contralateral femoral sheath to the neck of the aneurysm. The microcatheter is then advanced into the aneurysm dome while the balloon is uninflated. Finally, the balloon is carefully inflated so as to occlude the neck of the aneurysm, while the tip of the microcatheter is in a location in the body of the aneurysm that is suitable for detachable coil deposition. The balloon is temporarily inflated to obliterate the neck, and then the coil is delivered into the aneurysm. The balloon stabilizes the microcatheter in the aneurysm and prevents the coil mass herniation into

the parent artery. Furthermore, the balloon helps the coil to assume the 3-D shape of the aneurysm and allows adequate packing. After each coil is positioned but before detachment, the balloon is deflated to test the stability of the coil mass. The coil is detached if no displacement is observed; this process is repeated until the aneurysm had been adequately occluded. If movement of the coil is detected after balloon deflation, the coil is deemed not well anchored within the aneurysm and the coil is not detached.

This technique is usually most suitable for proximal aneurysms of the internal carotid artery (ICA), or the vertebrobasilar tree. However, it has been used for more distal aneurysms like anterior communicating artery aneurysms (Acom),[29,30] MCA aneurysms,[30] and posterior cerebral artery aneurysms.[30,31]

The application of this technique has been associated with complete angiographic obliteration in

77% to 83% of aneurysms.[30,32] However, the incidence of intraprocedural rupture with this technique can be as high as 5%, double that encountered with simple coiling.[30]

Moret and colleagues,[30] reported in their series that 20 of 21 totally occluded aneurysms remained totally occluded at follow-up angiography 3 to 6 months later.

Lefkowitz and colleagues[32] in their series of 23 aneurysms treated with the balloon-remodeling technique, no aneurysm required further treatment after a mean follow-up of 10 months. They were able to achieve complete occlusion of the aneurysm in 83% of the cases; the 17% remaining had an occlusion from 95% to 100% and 96% of the patients were at their neurologic baseline after the procedure. Aletich and colleagues[33] reported in their series of 75 aneurysms with a wide neck that they were able to apply the balloon-remodeling technique for 66 of them. Three failures were a result of tortuosity of the access vessels and four failures were a result of balloon inadequacies. They had a complete acute occlusion in 26% of the cases, subtotal (>95%) occlusion in 53%, and incomplete (<95%) occlusion in 21% of the cases. None of the aneurysms treated ruptured during the period of follow-up. In 5.1% of patients a permanent neurologic deficit was related to the procedure. The mortality rate related to the procedure was 3.8%.

Cottier and colleagues,[34] in their series of 49 balloon-assisted coilings, found a correlation between sac diameter and rate of occlusion. The larger the aneurysm the lower the possibility of dense packing in the sac and at the neck there was no statistical relationship between neck size and occlusion rate or between occlusion rate and the sac diameter/neck size ratio.

Ross and Dhillon[35] reported their experience with 50 cases treated with this technique and they defined a category of patients in whom this technique should not be applied: older patients, tortuous vessels, and distal aneurysms where it is difficult to place 2 microcatheters. They concluded that it is a technique achievable in most aneurysms allowing denser packing of the aneurysm while stabilizing the microcatheter.

Onyx HD 500

A new endovascular method is to fill the aneurysms with the liquid embolic agent Onyx HD 500 (Micro Therapeutics, Irvine, CA). Aneurysm treatment with Onyx in humans was introduced by Mawad and colleagues.[36] A prospective study (CAMEO trial) was conducted in 20 European centers and showed good results in selected patients with aneurysms that are unsuitable for coil treatment or in whom previous treatment has failed to occlude the aneurysm. Treatment morbidity was comparable to that of published prospective data on endovascular results for this subgroup of patients.[36–38] More follow-up and larger studies are needed to better evaluate this technique.

DECONSTRUCTIVE APPROACH

The deconstructive approach involves the occlusion of the parent vessel or several afferent vessels to the aneurysm. This results in thrombosis of the vessel-aneurysm complex. For prevention of ischemic events and stroke, a temporary test balloon occlusion should first be performed. Under careful cardiovascular and neurologic monitoring, the balloon is inflated into the parent vessel under normotensive conditions for a duration that varies from minutes to half an hour. If no changes are noted in the neurophysiological patient assessment, a hypotension challenge to two-thirds normal blood pressure is performed. The presence of adequate collateral blood flow to the parent vessel determines the outcome of the test. If the patient successfully passes all aspects of temporary balloon occlusion, permanent occlusion is performed usually immediately thereafter. However, if the patient shows neurologic changes during any aspect of the test, he or she is a candidate for surgical bypass before permanent vessel occlusion.

Permanent balloon occlusion is performed similar to temporary test occlusion. After careful selection of the appropriate balloon size, positioning through a microcatheter is performed. The target location is proximal to the aneurysm and may include the aneurysm neck. Balloon detachment is similar to coil detachment techniques. In some instances, prevention of balloon migration along the forces of cerebral blood flow is achieved by the use of two balloons in series.

POSTOPERATIVE CARE

Postoperative care is routinely performed initially in the postanesthesia care unit and then in the neurosurgical intensive care unit. All elective patients are hospitalized overnight with an average length of stay between 48 and 72 hours in our institution. Continuous cardiovascular monitoring and hourly neurologic examinations are performed for the first 24 hours. Heparin anticoagulation is maintained for 24 hours and at times followed by 24-hour dextran infusion for additional rheologic effects. The intra-arterial sheath is not removed during the first 24 hours for the possibility of emergent angiography or retreatment during the acute postoperative period. A Fem-Stop or other closure devices such as Angioseal or Duett can be used for successful arterial closure. A normal partial thromboplastin time (PTT) is recommended for these procedures to prevent local or retroperitoneal hematoma formation.

INTERVAL ANGIOGRAPHY AND FOLLOW-UP

Follow-up cerebral angiography and a gadolinium-enhanced magnetic resonance angiography (MRA) are routinely performed in 6 months. Thereafter, the patients are followed in 6-month intervals with MRA for the first 18 months.[17] The frequency of imaging by MRA is decreased to annual as long as there are no signs of recurrence. In that instance, the patient is scheduled for cerebral angiography.

Chronic anticoagulation is not required for routine embolization cases. Antiplatelet therapy with aspirin or clopidogrel bisulfate (Plavix) is most commonly used in patients with intra-arterial stents to prevent clotting and emboli formation. A 75-mg dose of Plavix every day is the preferred antiplatelet treatment in our institution.

COMPLICATIONS AND THEIR MANAGEMENT

The cause of endovascular complications is multifactorial and includes operator skills and experience; location, size, and morphology of the aneurysm; and presence of rupture. In most published series, the main complications include thromboembolic events and intraprocedural rupture.[27]

Thromboembolism

The rate of reported thromboembolic events varies widely from 2.5% to 28%.[39–44] The incidence of silent infarcts or infarcts causing transient ischemic attacks are demonstrated by magnetic resonance diffusion-weighted imaging and may be as high as 60% to 80%. The most common cause is catheter and coil manipulation and the incidence is higher in wide-neck aneurysms requiring assisting devices.[45–47] Two studies have shown that thromboembolic complications are more likely to occur in ACom and MCA aneurysms.[48] The complexity of the branching vessels off the parent artery and the poor visualization of these regions with routine angiography could explain such high incidence.

In our experience, the first and last coils play an instrumental role in avoidance of complications and careful techniques should be implemented in their deployment. Placement of the first coil should be made with as few attempts as possible to minimize disturbance of thrombi that may have formed either on the dome or the coil itself. The last coil should not be forced into the coil construct because damage of the parent vessel could provide a thrombogenic surface for future thromboembolic events.

Avoidance of such complications may be achieved by careful monitoring of the patient's response to heparin and by maintaining full anticoagulation levels during and following the procedure. If indeed part of the coil herniates into the parent vessel following deployment, then more extensive heparin anticoagulation is used postoperatively (average of 72 hours), followed by 24- to 48-hour dextran infusion and at least 6 weeks of antiplatelet therapy (aspirin or clopidogrel bisulfate). If the coil construct is not stable in the aneurysm dome, then a stent may be placed to wedge the construct into the aneurysm and prevent herniation into the parent vessel. If a thrombus is noted during the procedure, then the aneurysm should be secured by embolization in a timely fashion and intra-arterial thrombolysis may begin. The preferred agents for intra-arterial or intravenous thrombolysis are tissue plasminogen activator, urokinase, and abciximab. The use of IIb/IIIa inhibitors has been suggested as a safe and effective alternative by Fiorella and colleagues,[49] in a study that showed 100% complete or partial thrombus resolution without significant complications.

Intraprocedural Rupture

The reported incidence of intraprocedural rupture varies from 2% to 8% in patients treated with coil embolization.[18,20,50–52] In our institution, the incidence of intraprocedural rupture is 1.4% and most commonly occurs during the introduction of the microcatheter or guiding wire into the aneurysm and during coil delivery. Some noted risk factors for rupture are small size, history of recent rupture, and presence of a secondary sac.[17]

Operator experience is of paramount importance in prevention of such events. Raymond and Roy[51] demonstrated a progressive reduction in rupture incidence over the course of 3 years. In 75 treated patients, the incidence in the first 25 patients was 20%, in the next 25 patients 4%, and the remaining 25 patients did not have any complications. As mentioned earlier, careful placement of the first and last coils could prevent such complications. The choice of the first coil should minimize tension and stress against the aneurysm dome. Therefore, soft, hydrophilic coils are preferred and are usually undersized by

1 mm to 2 mm compared with the maximum dome diameter. The last coil should be placed without difficulty or significant force to prevent increases in tension across the fundus.

In a situation of intraprocedural rupture, it is important not to withdraw the offending device (microcatheter, guiding wire, or coils), as it acts as a plug at the rupture site. If the rupture occurs with a microcatheter or guiding wire, then delivery of a coil to decrease blood flow across the rupture site is recommended. Similarly, if the coil causes the rupture, then coil delivery should be completed. The goal is to secure the remainder of the aneurysm sac in a timely fashion and to reverse anticoagulation. Postoperatively, the patient should be closely monitored in the neurosurgical intensive care unit with frequent neurologic examinations and careful management of mean arterial blood pressure.

FUTURE DIRECTIONS

Although the annual risk of rebleeding from partially embolized or recurrent aneurysms is not well known, the rate of recanalization following endovascular aneurysm management remains a concern for treatment durability. Several modifications of bare platinum coils exist to increase the formation of thrombus within the aneurysm, thus reducing risk of recanalization. The Matrix coil involves a platinum coil with an outer coating of a bioabsorbable polymeric material (polyglycolic acid/lactide) that has been shown in swine aneurysm models to accelerate aneurysm fibrosis and neointima formation with increased neck tissue thickness but no parent artery stenosis.[53,54] The Cerecyte coil (Micrus) uses a similar polyglycolic acid material but as an inner coating of a platinum coil. A different bioactive coil technology, the Hydrogel coil (Microvention), consists of a platinum coil coated with a polymer that "swells" upon contact with blood increasing coil volume by a three- to ninefold. The clinical efficacy of these coils remains to be seen. The future of bioactive endovascular technology will likely involve delivery of growth factors (vascular endothelial growth factor, transforming growth factor-B, fibroblast growth factor), gene therapies, or cellular substrates within the aneurysm that will regenerate an endothelial wall layer across the aneurysm neck.[55–63]

SUMMARY

Data from our clinical series and others supports the idea that endovascular coil embolization is a reliable form of treatment for both ruptured and

---

Box 3
Jefferson Hospital for Neuroscience endovascular treatment protocol

- Placement arterial line, central venous line, and ventriculostomy for HH 3–4 in all SAH patients.
- General anesthesia
- Neurophysiological monitoring: baer (for posterior circulation and Pcom aneurysms), SSEP, EEG.
- MAP lowered 15% to 20% during coil deployment.
- Heparin 2000 units after "DOME" secured. - ACT 2.0–2.5X baseline, fresh ventriculostomy does not limit heparinization.
- Goal - no filling of aneurysm under full anti-coagulation - rotation in multiple views.
- MAP increased to 100 mm Hg after coiling completed to increase cerebral perfusion.
- Heparin infusion 24 hours with goal ACT 2X baseline followed by 24 hours dextran, anti-platelet agents when necessary.
- Follow-up angiography and MRA at 6 months.

---

unruptured cerebral aneurysms.[22,64–67] This form of treatment appears from preliminary data to be protective against subarachnoid hemorrhage.[22,65] Endovascular embolization in the current state of technological advancement carries acceptable morbidity and mortality when performed by experienced operators and is similar to that observed by other authors.[68] We have recently reported our 10-year experience of treating posterior circulation aneurysms with coil embolization in 236 patients harboring ruptured and unruptured aneurysms. To date this represents the largest series of posterior circulation aneurysms treated using coil embolization.[22,23,51,67,69,70] The International Subarachnoid Aneurysm Trial (ISAT) has reported that the relative risk of death or significant disability at 1 year for patients treated with coils was 22.6% lower than in surgically treated patients.[65] Treatment of cerebral aneurysms has to be determined on a case-by-case basis with primary emphasis given to patient comorbidities as well as the angioarchitecture of the aneurysm. The phenomenon of delayed reopening of coiled aneurysms is characterized in our experience by low incidence and a low rate of subsequent subarachnoid hemorrhage in patients followed for up to 5 years.[66,71]

Although not likely to replace open surgery, the continued advancements in technology and supportive clinical data will allow endovascular therapy to become a more durable mode of treatment. All patients should be evaluated by either a surgeon trained in both procedures or by an interventionalist and surgeon. The collaboration and amalgamation of this team approach benefits the patient and physician alike. Only future studies will delineate the long-term clinical and angiographic success of endosaccular therapy with the advent of covered stents, liquid embolic agents, and bioactive coils (**Box 3**).[72]

REFERENCES

1. Mettinger KL, Ericson K. Fibromuscular dysplasia and the brain. I. Observations on angiographic, clinical and genetic characteristics. Stroke 1982;13: 46–52.
2. Schievink WI, Katzmann JA, Piepgras DG. Alpha-1-antitrypsin deficiency in spontaneous intracranial arterial dissections. Cerebrovasc Dis 1998;8:42–4.
3. Schievink WI, Katzmann JA, Piepgras DG, et al. Alpha-1-antitrypsin phenotypes among patients with intracranial aneurysms. J Neurosurg 1996;84: 781–4.
4. Ruggieri PM, Poulos N, Masaryk TJ, et al. Occult intracranial aneurysms in polycystic kidney disease: screening with MR angiography. Radiology 1994; 191:33–9.
5. Wiebers DO, Whisnant JP, Huston J 3rd, et al. Unruptured intracranial aneurysms: natural history, clinical outcome, and risks of surgical and endovascular treatment. Lancet 2003;362:103–10.
6. Ljunggren B, Saveland H, Brandt L, et al. Early operation and overall outcome in aneurysmal subarachnoid hemorrhage. J Neurosurg 1985;62:547–51.
7. Whisnant JP, Sacco SE, O'Fallon WM, et al. Referral bias in aneurysmal subarachnoid hemorrhage. J Neurosurg 1993;78:726–32.
8. Hunt WE, Hess RM. Surgical risk as related to time of intervention in the repair of intracranial aneurysms. J Neurosurg 1968;28:14–20.
9. Guglielmi G, Vinuela F, Dion J, et al. Electrothrombosis of saccular aneurysms via endovascular approach. Part 2: preliminary clinical experience. J Neurosurg 1991;75:8–14.
10. Kassell NF, Torner JC, Haley EC Jr, et al. The International Cooperative Study on the Timing of Aneurysm Surgery. Part 1: overall management results. J Neurosurg 1990;73:18–36.
11. Kassell NF, Torner JC, Jane JA, et al. The International Cooperative Study on the Timing of Aneurysm Surgery. Part 2: surgical results. J Neurosurg 1990; 73:37–47.
12. Molyneux A, Kerr R, Stratton I, et al. International Subarachnoid Aneurysm Trial (ISAT) of neurosurgical clipping versus endovascular coiling in 2143 patients with ruptured intracranial aneurysms: a randomised trial. Lancet 2002;360:1267–74.
13. Butler P. Endovascular neurosurgery: a multidisciplinary approach. London: Springer; 2000.
14. Luo CB, Teng MM, Chang FC, et al. Endovascular embolization of ruptured cerebral aneurysms in patients older than 70 years. J Clin Neurosci 2007; 14:127–32.
15. Sugiura Y, Hiramatsu H, Miyamoto T, et al. Endovascular treatment of ruptured intracranial aneurysms using platinum coils in patients over 80 years of age. No Shinkei Geka 1999;27:147–54.
16. LeRoux Peter ND. Management of cerebral aneurysms. Philadelphia: Saunders; 2004.
17. Koebbe CJ, Veznedaroglu E, Jabbour P, et al. Endovascular management of intracranial aneurysms: current experience and future advances. Neurosurgery 2006;59:S93–102 [discussion: S103-113].
18. Vinuela F, Duckwiler G, Mawad M. Guglielmi detachable coil embolization of acute intracranial aneurysm: perioperative anatomical and clinical outcome in 403 patients. J Neurosurg 1997;86: 475–82.
19. Murayama Y, Nien YL, Duckwiler G, et al. Guglielmi detachable coil embolization of cerebral aneurysms: 11 years' experience. J Neurosurg 2003; 98:959–66.
20. Byrne JV, Sohn MJ, Molyneux AJ, et al. Five-year experience in using coil embolization for ruptured intracranial aneurysms: outcomes and incidence of late rebleeding. J Neurosurg 1999;90:656–63.
21. Raymond J, Guilbert F, Weill A, et al. Long-term angiographic recurrences after selective endovascular treatment of aneurysms with detachable coils. Stroke 2003;34:1398–403.
22. Eskridge JM, Song JK. Endovascular embolization of 150 basilar tip aneurysms with Guglielmi detachable coils: results of the Food and Drug Administration multicenter clinical trial. J Neurosurg 1998;89: 81–6.
23. Gruber DP, Zimmerman GA, Tomsick TA, et al. A comparison between endovascular and surgical management of basilar artery apex aneurysms. J Neurosurg 1999;90:868–74.
24. Thornton J, Debrun GM, Aletich VA, et al. Follow-up angiography of intracranial aneurysms treated with endovascular placement of Guglielmi detachable coils. Neurosurgery 2002;50:239–49 [discussion: 249–50].
25. Koivisto T, Vanninen R, Hurskainen H, et al. Outcomes of early endovascular versus surgical treatment of ruptured cerebral aneurysms. A prospective randomized study. Stroke 2000;31: 2369–77.
26. Harbaugh RE, Heros RC, Hadley MN. More on ISAT. Lancet 2003;361:783–4 [author reply 784].
27. Connors J. Strategies and practical techniques, in interventional neuroradiology. Philadelphia: Saunders; 1999.

28. Jabbour P, Koebbe C, Veznedaroglu E, et al. Stent-assisted coil placement for unruptured cerebral aneurysms. Neurosurg Focus 2004;17:E10.

29. Levy DI. Embolization of wide-necked anterior communicating artery aneurysm: technical note. Neurosurgery 1997;41:979–82.

30. Moret J, Cognard C, Weill A, et al. Reconstruction technic in the treatment of wide-neck intracranial aneurysms. Long-term angiographic and clinical results. Apropos of 56 cases. J Neuroradiol 1997; 24:30–44.

31. Mericle RA, Wakhloo AK, Rodriguez R, et al. Temporary balloon protection as an adjunct to endosaccular coiling of wide-necked cerebral aneurysms: technical note. Neurosurgery 1997; 41:975–8.

32. Lefkowitz MA, Gobin YP, Akiba Y, et al. Balloon-assisted Guglielmi detachable coiling of wide-necked aneurysma: part II–clinical results. Neurosurgery 1999;45:531–7 [discussion: 537–8].

33. Aletich VA, Debrun GM, Misra M, et al. The remodeling technique of balloon-assisted Guglielmi detachable coil placement in wide-necked aneurysms: experience at the University of Illinois at Chicago. J Neurosurg 2000;93:388–96.

34. Cottier JP, Pasco A, Gallas S, et al. Utility of balloon-assisted Guglielmi detachable coiling in the treatment of 49 cerebral aneurysms: a retrospective, multicenter study. AJNR Am J Neuroradiol 2001; 22:345–51.

35. Ross IB, Dhillon GS. Balloon assistance as a routine adjunct to the endovascular treatment of cerebral aneurysms. Surg Neurol 2006;66:593–601 [discussion: 601–2].

36. Mawad ME, Cekirge S, Ciceri E, et al. Endovascular treatment of giant and large intracranial aneurysms by using a combination of stent placement and liquid polymer injection. J Neurosurg 2002;96: 474–82.

37. Molyneux AJ, Cekirge S, Saatci I, et al. Cerebral Aneurysm Multicenter European Onyx (CAMEO) trial: results of a prospective observational study in 20 European centers. AJNR Am J Neuroradiol 2004;25:39–51.

38. Weber W, Siekmann R, Kis B, et al. Treatment and follow-up of 22 unruptured wide-necked intracranial aneurysms of the internal carotid artery with Onyx HD 500. AJNR Am J Neuroradiol 2005;26:1909–15.

39. Alexander MJ, Duckwiler GR, Gobin YP, et al. Management of intraprocedural arterial thrombus in cerebral aneurysm embolization with abciximab: technical case report. Neurosurgery 2002;50: 899–901 [discussion: 901–2].

40. Cognard C, Pierot L, Boulin A, et al. Intracranial aneurysms: endovascular treatment with mechanical detachable spirals in 60 aneurysms. Radiology 1997;202:783–92.

41. Debrun GM, Aletich VA, Kehrli P, et al. Selection of cerebral aneurysms for treatment using Guglielmi detachable coils: the preliminary University of Illinois at Chicago experience. Neurosurgery 1998;43: 1281–95 [discussion: 1296–7].

42. Fessler RD, Ringer AJ, Qureshi AI, et al. Intracranial stent placement to trap an extruded coil during endovascular aneurysm treatment: technical note. Neurosurgery 2000;46:248–51 [discussion: 251–3].

43. Pelz DM, Lownie SP, Fox AJ. Thromboembolic events associated with the treatment of cerebral aneurysms with Guglielmi detachable coils. AJNR Am J Neuroradiol 1998;19:1541–7.

44. Qureshi AI, Mohammad Y, Yahia AM, et al. Ischemic events associated with unruptured intracranial aneurysms: multicenter clinical study and review of the literature. Neurosurgery 2000;46:282–9 [discussion: 289–290].

45. Rordorf G, Bellon RJ, Budzik RE Jr, et al. Silent thromboembolic events associated with the treatment of unruptured cerebral aneurysms by use of Guglielmi detachable coils: prospective study applying diffusion-weighted imaging. AJNR Am J Neuroradiol 2001;22:5–10.

46. Soeda A, Sakai N, Murao K, et al. Thromboembolic events associated with Guglielmi detachable coil embolization with use of diffusion-weighted MR imaging. Part II. Detection of the microemboli proximal to cerebral aneurysm. AJNR Am J Neuroradiol 2003;24:2035–8.

47. Soeda A, Sakai N, Sakai H, et al. Thromboembolic events associated with Guglielmi detachable coil embolization of asymptomatic cerebral aneurysms: evaluation of 66 consecutive cases with use of diffusion-weighted MR imaging. AJNR Am J Neuroradiol 2003;24:127–32.

48. Cronqvist M, Pierot L, Boulin A, et al. Local intraarterial fibrinolysis of thromboemboli occurring during endovascular treatment of intracerebral aneurysm: a comparison of anatomic results and clinical outcome. AJNR Am J Neuroradiol 1998;19:157–65.

49. Fiorella D, Albuquerque FC, Han P, et al. Strategies for the management of intraprocedural thromboembolic complications with abciximab (ReoPro). Neurosurgery 2004;54:1089–97 [discussion: 1097–8].

50. McDougall CG, Halbach VV, Dowd CF, et al. Causes and management of aneurysmal hemorrhage occurring during embolization with Guglielmi detachable coils. J Neurosurg 1998;89:87–92.

51. Raymond J, Roy D. Safety and efficacy of endovascular treatment of acutely ruptured aneurysms. Neurosurgery 1997;41:1235–45 [discussion: 1245–6].

52. Ricolfi F, Le Guerinel C, Blustajn J, et al. Rupture during treatment of recently ruptured aneurysms with Guglielmi electrodetachable coils. AJNR Am J Neuroradiol 1998;19:1653–8.

53. Murayama Y, Tateshima S, Gonzalez NR, et al. Matrix and bioabsorbable polymeric coils accelerate healing of intracranial aneurysms: long-term experimental study. Stroke 2003;34:2031–7.
54. Murayama Y, Vinuela F, Tateshima S, et al. Bioabsorbable polymeric material coils for embolization of intracranial aneurysms: a preliminary experimental study. J Neurosurg 2001;94:454–63.
55. Abrahams JM, Diamond SL, Hurst RW, et al. Topic review: surface modifications enhancing biological activity of Guglielmi detachable coils in treating intracranial aneurysms. Surg Neurol 2000;54:34–40 [discussion: 40–1].
56. Abrahams JM, Forman MS, Grady MS, et al. Delivery of human vascular endothelial growth factor with platinum coils enhances wall thickening and coil impregnation in a rat aneurysm model. AJNR Am J Neuroradiol 2001;22:1410–7.
57. Abrahams JM, Song C, DeFelice S, et al. Endovascular microcoil gene delivery using immobilized anti-adenovirus antibody for vector tethering. Stroke 2002;33:1376–82.
58. de Gast AN, Altes TA, Marx WF, et al. Transforming growth factor beta-coated platinum coils for endovascular treatment of aneurysms: an animal study. Neurosurgery 2001;49:690–4 [discussion: 694–6].
59. Kallmes DF, Williams AD, Cloft HJ, et al. Platinum coil-mediated implantation of growth factor-secreting endovascular tissue grafts: an in vivo study. Radiology 1998;207:519–23.
60. Kawakami O, Miyamoto S, Hatano T, et al. Accelerated embolization healing of aneurysms by polyethylene terephthalate coils seeded with autologous fibroblasts. Neurosurgery 2005;56:1075–81 [discussion: 1075–81].
61. Marx WE, Cloft HJ, Helm GA, et al. Endovascular treatment of experimental aneurysms by use of biologically modified embolic devices: coil-mediated intraaneurysmal delivery of fibroblast tissue allografts. AJNR Am J Neuroradiol 2001;22:323–33.
62. Matsumoto H, Terada T, Tsuura M, et al. Basic fibroblast growth factor released from a platinum coil with a polyvinyl alcohol core enhances cellular proliferation and vascular wall thickness: an in vitro and in vivo study. Neurosurgery 2003;53:402–7 [discussion: 407–8].
63. Ohyama T, Nishide T, Iwata H, et al. Immobilization of basic fibroblast growth factor on a platinum microcoil to enhance tissue organization in intracranial aneurysms. J Neurosurg 2005;102:109–15.
64. Evans JJ, Sekhar LN, Rak R, et al. Bypass grafting and revascularization in the management of posterior circulation aneurysms. Neurosurgery 2004;55:1036–49.
65. Molyneux AJ, Kerr RS, Yu LM, et al. International Subarachnoid Aneurysm Trial (ISAT) of neurosurgical clipping versus endovascular coiling in 2143 patients with ruptured intracranial aneurysms: a randomised comparison of effects on survival, dependency, seizures, rebleeding, subgroups, and aneurysm occlusion. Lancet 2005;366:809–17.
66. Pandey AS, Koebbe C, Rosenwasser RH, et al. Endovascular coil embolization of ruptured and unruptured posterior circulation aneurysms: review of a 10-year experience. Neurosurgery 2007;60:626–36 [discussion: 636–7].
67. Pierot L, Boulin A, Castaings L, et al. Endovascular treatment of pericallosal artery aneurysms. Neurol Res 1996;18:49–53.
68. Leibowitz R, Do HM, Marcellus ML, et al. Parent vessel occlusion for vertebrobasilar fusiform and dissecting aneurysms. AJNR Am J Neuroradiol 2003;24:902–7.
69. Bendok BR, Przybylo JH, Parkinson R, et al. Neuroendovascular interventions for intracranial posterior circulation disease via the transradial approach: technical case report. Neurosurgery 2005;56:E626 [discussion: E626].
70. Lempert TE, Malek AM, Halbach VV, et al. Endovascular treatment of ruptured posterior circulation cerebral aneurysms. Clinical and angiographic outcomes. Stroke 2000;31:100–10.
71. Pandey A, Rosenwasser RH, Veznedaroglu E. Management of distal anterior cerebral artery aneurysms: a single institution retrospective analysis (1997–2005). Neurosurgery 2007;61:909–16 [discussion: 916–7].
72. Veznedaroglu E, Koebbe CJ, Siddiqui A, et al. Initial experience with bioactive cerecyte detachable coils: impact on reducing recurrence rates. Neurosurgery 2008;62:799–805 [discussion: 805–6].

Endovascular Treatment of Intracranial Arteriovenous Malformation

Dorothea Strozyk, MD[a,b], Raul G. Nogueira, MD[c], Sean D. Lavine, MD[a,b],*

KEYWORDS

- Arteriovenous malformation • Endovascular treatment
- Intracranial hemorrhage • Embolization • NBCA • Onyx

Arteriovenous malformations (AVMs) of the brain are vascular lesions in which an abnormal tangle or nidus of vessels permits pathologic shunting of blood flow from the arterial to the venous tree without an intervening capillary bed. AVMs typically present in young adults (mean 35 years ±SD 18)[1] and have a variety of clinical manifestations including most commonly hemorrhage, but also seizures, headaches, and progressive neurologic deterioration.[2] Since the advent of contemporary brain imaging techniques, an increasing number of AVMs are detected before they hemorrhage. The number of AVMs identified before rupture is now twice those identified after rupture. This has led to new considerations and modifications of interdisciplinary AVM management strategies.[3]

The ultimate goal of AVM therapy is complete obliteration of the lesion because any residual AVM might result in hemorrhage and partial treatment may increase the chances of bleeding.[4–6] Complete obliteration is more commonly achieved by multimodal therapy rather than by embolization alone. The available options for treatment include endovascular embolization, microsurgical resection, radiosurgery, medical management, or a combination of these treatment modalities.

Neuroendovascular therapy is a critical component of this multidisciplinary and multimodal approach. In general, because the risk of rebleeding is high, and the main cause of disability in patients with AVMs is hemorrhage, early assessment and delineation of a stepwise treatment plan is recommended for those who have experienced an AVM-related intracranial hemorrhage (ICH). Newer embolization techniques and embolic agents will continue to be developed and introduced, affecting the treatments associated with embolization. Although better techniques allow a more aggressive embolization of the AVM nidus, it is unclear at this time if some portion of the complication risks previously carried by surgical resection may be transferred to the embolization procedure.

EPIDEMIOLOGY

The incidence and prevalence of intracranial AVMs has been mainly estimated from autopsy series and retrospective population-based studies. In the Cooperative Study of Intracranial Aneurysms and Subarachnoid Hemorrhage, symptomatic AVMs were found in 8.6% of all nontraumatic subarachnoid hemorrhages.[7]

During the era before noninvasive brain imaging, one autopsy series detected a prevalence of 4.3%.[8] Although not derived from a population-based study, these data are of interest because

[a] Department of Neurosurgery, Columbia University, College of Physicians and Surgeons, New York, NY, USA
[b] Department of Radiology, Columbia University, College of Physicians and Surgeons, New York, NY, USA
[c] Department of Neurology, Massachusetts General Hospital/Harvard Medical School, MGH-55 Fruit Street, Blake 12-Room 1291, Boston, MA 02114, USA
* Corresponding author. Endovascular Neurosurgery, Columbia University Medical Center, 710 West 168th Street, Neurological Institute 4th Floor 424, New York, NY 10032.
E-mail address: S12081@columbia.edu (S.D. Lavine).

Neurosurg Clin N Am 20 (2009) 399–418
doi:10.1016/j.nec.2009.07.004
1042-3680/09/$ – see front matter © 2009 Published by Elsevier Inc.

they represent a careful autopsy-based effort to determine the prevalence of AVMs.

In the Netherlands Antilles, between 1980 and 1990, an annual incidence of 1.1 symptomatic AVMs per 100,000 people was identified.[9] In this fairly isolated and homogenous population, however, an unusually high proportion of the patients had multiple brain AVMs (25%) and hereditary hemorrhagic teleangiectesia, or Rendu-Osler-Weber disease (35%), making it difficult to compare the findings with those described in other populations.

In a retrospective, population-based study conducted over 27 years in Olmsted County, Minnesota, the incidence of symptomatic ICH due to any type of intracranial vascular malformations was 0.8 per 100,000.[10,11] Over many years, the Olmsted County study has provided the most reliable data concerning the detection rate of brain AVMs. A limitation of the study is its relatively small and homogenous population base, and conclusions drawn for AVMs were based on only few lesions detected between 1965 and 1992.

The New York Islands Arteriovenous Malformation Study is the first ongoing prospective population-based survey determining the incidence of AVM hemorrhage and associated morbidity and mortality rates in a population of more than 9 million people located in New York. Initial results calculated an AVM detection rate of 1.34 per 100,000 person years and a first-ever acute AVM hemorrhage rate of 0.51 per 100,000 person-years.[1] These rates reflect increased use of MRI due to low threshold for imaging. As many as 62% of the AVMs in this study were diagnosed before hemorrhage.

PATHOGENESIS

Most brain AVMs occur sporadically; however, they also have been associated with several congenital and hereditary syndromes, including Rendu-Osler-Weber disease (hereditary hemorrhagic teleangiectesia), Wyburn-Mason syndrome, and Sturge-Weber disease.[12–14] Rare familial cases not associated with syndromes also have been described.[15]

Recent evidence suggests that not all brain AVMs are congenital in origin.[16] Although the large majority probably occur congenitally due to failure of capillary formation during early embryogenesis,[17] some AVMs seem to form in response to a postnatal stimulus of angiogenesis, particularly in younger patients. De novo development of AVMs in children and in adults has been reported.[18,19] Moreover, AVMs have reoccurred in children after complete surgical resection.[20]

CLINICAL PRESENTATION

ICH is the initial manifestation of AVMs in at least 50% of cases.[1,10,21,22] The next most common presentation is seizure, which occurs in approximately one third of cases, often alerting a physician to the presence of an AVM.[23–25] The available literature documents a remarkable variation in incidence of seizures associated with AVMs. Inconsistent data from reports preclude accurate determination of the relationship between seizures and subsequent risk of ICH. Several types of attacks labeled as seizures occur, and the type of seizure is often unreported in studies.

Headache is the presenting symptom in approximately 15% of AVM patients. Because headaches are a common complaint in the population at large, it is difficult to determine if the headaches associated with AVMs are unique to the condition. In contrast to early assumptions, the headaches in AVMs are of no distinctive type, frequency, persistence, or severity. Migraine headaches with and without aura have been documented in the literature.[26] Little evidence supports the claim that recurrent unilateral headaches should arouse suspicion of an ipsilateral AVM. The yield for AVMs in evaluation for headache is low; in one study, only 0.2% of patients with normal neurologic findings who underwent neuroimaging for headache were diagnosed with AVM.[27] The postoperative disappearance of migraine headaches is not unusual and may occur after any type of operation.

Focal neurologic signs without hemorrhage are distinctively rare. Slowly progressing neurologic deficits, once considered common, are part of the presentation in only few patients (4% to 8%).[28–32] Shunting through a low resistance AVM results in hypoperfusion of the surrounding normal brain tissue, a phenomenon known as "vascular steal"; however, evidence for a causal link with ischemic symptoms is lacking.[24] Venous hypertension and mass effect of the nidus offer alternative explanations for progressing focal neurologic deficits.[33]

NATURAL HISTORY

The risks of invasive management should be evaluated against the background of the natural history of the disease. Ideally, physicians need to know whether or not there are large numbers of relatively asymptomatic patients who live normal lives; whether or not nonhemorrhagic but symptomatic patients can be maintained with conservative therapy only; and whether or not patients who have hemorrhaged in the past are prone to hemorrhage again.

Unfortunately, little unbiased natural history data are available, in part, because brain AVMs are rare and heterogenous and also because most undergo some form of treatment. The natural history of AVMs is variable depending on patient characteristics, duration of follow-up, treatments used, and ascertainment of endpoints. Most series have retrospectively collected data, usually with limited follow-up periods, often lacking consistent angiographic assessment, and focusing on non-operable lesions, causing a bias toward AVMs that are larger, deeper, or located in eloquent areas of the brain.

Notwithstanding these shortcomings, once an AVM has been detected, for one reason or another, a reasonable overall estimate of the annual risk of bleeding is 2% to 4%.[23,34–36] In the year immediately after a symptomatic hemorrhage, the rehemorrhage risk is generally thought considerably higher, approximately 6%[37,38] to 18%[39,40] for the first year, gradually returning toward the 2% to 4% baseline with time.[35,41]

Graf and colleagues[38] reviewed the records of 191 patients with AVMs with a mean period of follow-up of 2 to 5 years. They found a high rate of initial ICH in the age group 11 to 35 years old, and the rate of rebleeding was approximately 2% per year. Smaller lesions were more prone to ICH, and approximately 13% of the patients died as a result of the hemorrhage. Asymptomatic hemorrhages may not come to medical attention leading to underreporting in bleeding rates. One study has shown that approximately 15% of operated AVMs show evidence of prior asymptomatic hemorrhage.[42]

Risk factors for hemorrhage identified by more than one study and, therefore, not likely to represent a chance finding, include history of prior hemorrhage,[40,43,44] exclusive deep venous drainage,[45–47] presence of a single draining vein,[43,48] high intranidal pressures,[45,49,50] and the presence of intranidal aneurysms.[51,52] The relevance of these risk factors was recently reported by Stapf and colleagues. These investigators analyzed follow-up data on 622 consecutive patients from the prospective Columbia AVM database, limited to the period between initial AVM diagnosis and the start of treatment (ie, any endovascular, surgical, or radiation therapy). The mean pretreatment follow-up was 829 days (median: 102 days) during which 39 (6%) patients experienced AVM hemorrhage. Increasing age (hazard ratio [HR] 1.05; 95% CI, 1.03–1.08), initial hemorrhagic AVM presentation (HR 5.38; 95% CI, 2.64–10.96), deep brain location (HR 3.25; 95% CI, 1.30–8.16), and exclusive deep venous drainage (HR 3.25; 95% CI, 1.01–5.67) were independent predictors of subsequent hemorrhage. Annual hemorrhage rates on follow-up ranged from 0.9% for patients without hemorrhagic AVM presentation, deep AVM location, or deep venous drainage to as high as 34.4% for those harboring all three risk factors.[53]

The reported long-term annual mortality rates are 1% to 1.5%.[36,54] Long-term mortality is increased in untreated AVM in particular in male patients, and can be reduced with active treatment.[55] An estimated 10% to 30% of survivors have long-term disability.[41]

GRADING

A widely used method to predict the risk of morbidity and mortality attending the operative treatment of AVMs is the Spetzler-Martin grading system (**Table 1**). The total grade reflects the sum of points assigned for nidus size (<3 cm, 3–6 cm, >6 cm), eloquence of adjacent brain, and pattern

Table 1
Classification of arteriovenous malformations as proposed by Spetzler and Martin

Arteriovenous Malformation Characteristics	Grading
Size of the arteriovenous malformation	
o Small (<3 cm)	1 point
o Medium (3–6 cm)	2 points
o Large (>6 cm)	3 points
Localization of the arteriovenous malformation	
o Noneloquent	0 point
o Eloquent	1 point
Venous drainage	
o Only superficial	0 point
o Deep	1 point

Data from Spetzler RF, Martin NA. A proposed grading system for arteriovenous malformations. J Neurosurg 1986;65:476–83.

of venous drainage (deep versus superficial). If any or all of the venous drainage egressed through deep veins (internal cerebral, basal veins, precentral cerebellar vein), it was categorized as deep. An AVM was considered adjacent to eloquent brain parenchyma if it was next to the sensorimotor cortex, language areas, visual cortex, hypothalamus, thalamus, internal capsule, brainstem, cerebellar peduncles, or deep cerebellar nuclei. Spetzler-Martin grades range from I to V summing the points for each category. A separate grade VI is reserved for inoperable lesions.

The Spetzler-Martin grading system was originally developed to predict the perioperative and postsurgical outcome and, as such, has shown a reliable correlation with surgical outcome.[56] Although many other grading scales have been proposed,[57–60] all of which focus on anatomic, hemodynamic, and physiologic properties of the AVM, the Spetzler-Martin grading scale has become the scale used most often by treating physicians.

In general, Spetzler-Martin AVM grades I, II, or III were found to have low treatment-associated morbidity (1% to 3%) but much higher morbidity rates were observed for grade IV and V lesions, reaching 31% and 50%, respectively, in the early postoperative period. In addition, the rate for permanent deficit was 29.9% for grade IV lesions and 16.7% for grade V lesions.[61] A similar relationship between Spetzler-Martin scale and outcome was observed by Heros and colleagues.[62]

To date, these data form the foundation for most management decisions regarding AVM therapy. Operative morbidity and mortality rates for grade I and II AVMs are approximately 1%. These lesions are generally resected, because the risk of hemorrhage far outweighs the risk for surgical resection. In such lesions, preoperative embolization is not frequently pursued, given that the risk of the embolization procedure may approach or even surpass the risk of surgery. In highly eloquent brain regions, stereotactic radiosurgery rather than surgical resection may be pursued. The role for curative embolization of these low-grade AVMs has yet to be evaluated in a systematic basis and compared with these surgical results.

The operative morbidity and mortality rate for a grade III AVM is 3%, although this is probably more accurate for small-sized grade III AVMs. Larger grade III and those in eloquent brain areas (with or without deep drainage) may carry a higher combined surgical morbidity and mortality risk.[63] This complex and heterogenous group requires an individualized assessment on a case-by-case basis. Most of these lesions are treated with radiosurgery or preoperative embolization followed by surgical resection.

The surgical resection of grade IV and V AVMs is generally associated with a risk of operative morbidity and mortality that exceeds the risks associated with the natural history of the lesion.[4] In addition, in this group of patients, partial AVM treatment substantially increased the yearly risk for hemorrhage. In accordance with these observations, surgical treatment for grade IV and V AVMs is recommended only in patients with progressive neurologic deficits attributable to repeated hemorrhage or disabling symptoms, such as intractable seizures.

Although the Spetzler-Martin grading scale was designed to predict surgical outcome, it has also been evaluated in the combined management of AVMs, including surgical resection, embolization followed by surgical resection, embolization alone, or radiosurgery.[64] Deterioration due to treatment was seen in 19% of patients with grade I or II AVMs, 35% of patients with grade III lesions, and 42% of patients with grade IV or V lesions. The scale does not include characteristics, such as associated aneurysms, venous stasis, or venous aneurysms, that have been associated with hemorrhagic risk. There are no reliable data, in fact, correlating such features with treatment risk.

DIAGNOSIS

Intracranial AVMs may be diagnosed with a variety of diagnostic noninvasive imaging studies, including CT and CT angiography. Noninvasive conventional and functional MRI techniques are playing an increasing role in the interventional management because they facilitate localization of the nidus in relation to the brain and further identify functionally important brain areas adjacent to the nidus.[65,66]

Nevertheless, catheter angiography remains the gold standard for defining the arterial and venous anatomy.[67] Confidence in the diagnosis of AVMs is crucial in planning the appropriate therapy. Brain AVMs must be separated from other intracranial AV fistulas, which at times have similar morphologic features on conventional imaging studies. These lesions, however, differ in terms of pathogenesis, natural course, and treatment strategies.

A diagnostic angiogram studying an AVM should provide detailed information regarding the number of feeding arteries and their vascular territories and delineate the venous drainage. This information is usually sufficient to estimate the number of stages required for adequate presurgical embolization.

Hemodynamic effects due to shunting cause an opening of collateral vessels in territories adjacent to but not primarily involved in the AVM. Collateral vessels that are enlarged because of hemodynamic effects can be prominently seen during angiography and can be easily misinterpreted as being part of the nidus. Such collateral vessels are sometimes referred to as areas of angiomatous change.[68] It is important during angiographic analysis of an AVM to differentiate the tortuous, often bizarre appearance of such collateral vessels from the primary nidus. Additionally, a dysplastic appearance is frequently seen in the angiographic behavior of feeding pedicles in an AVM. This morphologic change is termed, "flow-induced angiopathy."[69]

The angiographic images should be evaluated carefully for the presence of aneurysms. Because of their propensity for hemorrhage, aneurysms should generally be addressed before the remainder of the lesion. These aneurysms may be located on vessels that are remote from the nidus, on a feeding vessel—so-called flow-related aneurysms, or within the nidus itself, termed "intranidal aneurysms."

Flow phenomena associated with the AVM provide a logical mechanism to explain the greater than expected prevalence of aneurysms on AVM feeding vessels. No histologic or imaging features have been found to distinguish flow-related aneurysms occurring in association with AVMs from those aneurysms occurring in absence of AVMs. Redekop and colleagues[51] found 11.2% of aneurysms of AVMs, whereas aneurysms on vessels unrelated to the AVM were found in only 0.8%.

Controversy surrounds the origin of intranidal aneurysms (Fig. 1). Many believe that these lesions represent true aneurysms located in the most distal arterial branches adjacent to the AVM nidus. Others have suggested, however, that some of these lesions represent early filling of dilated venous pouches rather than true arterial aneurysms or may even represent pseudoaneurysms arising as residua of prior hemorrhages.[70] On conventional angiographic views, intranidal aneurysms may be occasionally obscured by overlying vessels or other portions of the AVM nidus. Thus, when one or more AVM-related hemorrhages are observed in patients with unresectable AVMs, endovascular exploration with superselective angiography represents a reasonable strategy.

The venous phase images represent another critical component of the angiographic evaluation. The visualization of draining veins can vary with the parent vessel injected because different parts of the nidus are opacified and are associated with patterns of contrast washout. The presence of any pre-existing venous outflow stenoses should be noted because inadvertent occlusion of venous efflux during embolization represents one of the most dangerous complications that may be encountered.

In many cases, rapid AV shunting superimposes the arterial feeders, the nidus, and the draining veins, obscuring important features, such as small arterial feeders, distal feeding pedicles, nidal aneurysms, direct AV fistulas, and small accessory draining veins. Hence, superselective angiography is often needed to ascertain the finer details of the AVM using microcatheters advanced into distal aspects of the arterial feeders.[71] Superselective angiography may often be combined with endovascular treatment of these lesions.

TREATMENT

Therapeutic management of AVMs requires a careful multidisciplinary approach to estimate a risk-to-benefit ratio for individual patients. All patients should be evaluated by physicians who have expertise in endovascular embolization, surgical resection, and radiosurgery. The balance between benefits and risks of any form of treatment (surgical excision, endovascular embolization, or radiosurgery) has never been assessed in randomized controlled trials; hence, selecting therapeutic options can be challenging. A randomized trial of unruptured brain AVMs (ARUBA) compairing endovascular treatment, surgery or radiosurgery to medical treatment is currently underway.

The role of endovascular management can be summarized in five scenarios[72]:

1. Preoperative: embolization as a precursor to complete curative surgical resection
2. Preradiosurgery: embolization as a precursor to radiation therapy
3. Targeted therapy: embolization to eradicate a specific bleeding source

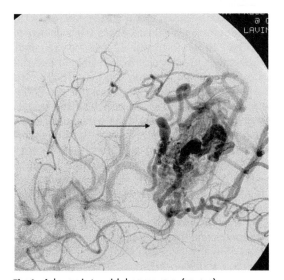

Fig. 1. A large intranidal aneurysm (arrow).

4. Curative: embolization for attempted cure
5. Palliative: embolization to palliate symptoms attributed to shunting

Preoperative Embolization

AVM embolization is most commonly performed as a precursor to surgical resection, although many small, superficial brain AVMs can be surgically resected without preoperative embolization with minimal morbidity and mortality. In these cases, the additional risks of embolization may not be justified. There are, however, exceptions, such as grade I and II AVMs with a deep arterial feeding artery that are difficult to access surgically. Embolization is used frequently for Spetzler-Martin grade III AVMs, particularly for those in central and eloquent locations and those with deep feeders. Preoperative embolization is also commonly done for Spetzler-Martin grades IV and V AVMs.[73]

Studies comparing surgery with and without embolization do not exist in a prospectively controlled fashion; nevertheless, several case series have demonstrated that preoperative embolization results in improvements in overall treatment outcomes. Advantages include diminished blood loss and shorter surgical times by decreasing the size of the nidus and the amount of blood flow through the AVM.[74] Embolized vessels are also more readily identified during surgery and can provide a road map for the resection of the arterial feeders and nidus while preserving en passage arteries to nearby eloquent parenchyma. Finally, staged flow reduction in the nidus can decrease the incidence of potentially catastrophic hemorrhage.[75–77]

In a series of patients treated with combined endovascular and surgical interventions, morbidity resulting from preoperative endovascular embolization was classified as mild in 3.9% of the cases, moderate in 6.9%, and severe in 1.98%.[78] Morgan and colleagues[79] described a 33% total complication rate in their predominantly surgical series, which included only 18% preoperative embolizations. The data were not presented separately for ruptured and unruptured cases.

In the Columbia Presbyterian AVM series, 119 AVM patients were followed prospectively after treatment. Treatment-related nondisabling neurologic deficits were found in 50 patients (42%), resulting from surgery in 32%, embolization in 6%, and both treatment types in 4%. Another six patients had persistant disabling deficits (3% from surgery and 2% from embolization).[80] The most striking figures, however, are seen when treatment outcome is analyzed separately for ruptured and unruptured AVM cases. Among patients who initially presented with ICH, only 27% experienced new treatment-related deficits. By comparison, among patients diagnosed with an unruptured AVM, 58% experienced new treatment-related deficits. Hence, the risk of new treatment-related deficits in patients with a nonhemorrhagic presentation seems significantly higher than for patients after initial rupture. These observational data raise concerns that embolization of unruptured AVMs may increase the risk of symptomatic ICH and the onset of an acute, disabling, persisting clinical syndrome.

The efficacy of modern AVM embolization using N-butyl-cyanoacrylate (NBCA) in converting high Spetzler-Martin grade lesions to lower-grade lesions, with a concurrent reduction in morbidity and mortality, has been demonstrated in several clinical studies.[75,81] One randomized controlled trial intended to test equivalence between the embolic agents NBCA and polyvinyl alcohol (PVA) particles for the preoperative embolization of brain AVMs.[82] The primary outcome was the degree of vascular occlusion achieved as judged by the percent nidus reduction and number of feeding vessels treated on catheter angiography, and secondary outcomes were the duration of subsequent surgical resection and the number of transfusions required during surgery. The reduction of AVM dimensions (79.4% in the NBCA group and 86.9% in the PVA group) and the mean number of vessels embolized (2.2 in the NBCA group and 2.1 in the PVA group) were similar in the two groups. There was no difference in secondary outcomes except for more postresection ICHs in the PVA group (5% vs 17%, $P<.05$).

Preradiosurgery Embolization

The success of radiotherapy is inversely related to the size of the AVM nidus.[83] AVMs with a volume of less than 10 mL (diameter <3 cm) are frequently suitable for radiosurgery, with estimated rates of cure at 2 years ranging between 80% and 88%.[84,85] Hence, one of the major goals of endovascular therapy is to shrink the nidus into a smaller single target. Other goals include the treatment of nidal aneurysms that represent a risk for hemorrhage until the radiosurgically induced obliteration occurs and to attempt to obliterate large arteriovenous fistulae that are typically more refractory to the effects of radiosurgery. The major disadvantage of radiation therapy is a persistent risk of ICH, which may be as high as 10% until the lesion disappears and may persist even after obliteration of the AVM.[86,87] Possible adverse effects include extended radiation necrosis, intracranial arterial stenosis, and cranial nerve injury and are more likely to occur with increasing radiation dose, in patients with deep AVM location, and those who experience AVM rupture.

Gobin and colleagues described their experience with 125 patients who underwent embolization as a precursor to radiosurgery. Embolization produced total obliteration in 11.2% of AVMs and reduced 76% of AVMs enough to allow radiosurgery. Almost 90% of the AVMs with diameters between 4 and 6 cm, and less than 50% with diameters greater than 6 cm, had sufficient nidal size reduction for subsequent radiosurgery. Therefore, adjunctive embolization was most effective for AVMs 4 to 6 cm in diameter. There was no convincing advantage for combined embolization and radiosurgery compared with radiosurgery alone for AVMs smaller than 4 cm. Overall, embolization, and radiosurgery together produced total obliteration in 65% of the partially embolized AVMs.[88] More recently, Henkes and colleagues reported "total" obliteration in only 47% of patients undergoing combined embolization and radiosurgery. Most of the treated AVMs were of very high grade, possibly explaining the lower "total" obliteration rates.[89]

The absence of residual AVM nidus or AV shunting after radiosurgery does not equate with definite evidence of permanent obliteration of the AVM. Although a negative angiogram had been considered the practical endpoint defining successful treatment, a recent retrospective review of 236 radiosurgery-treated AVMs followed for a median of 6.4 years after angiographic evidence of obliteration found four cases of subsequent hemorrhage in the previous AVM site. Two cases were resected and found to have small regions of tiny patent AVM vessels. In each case, there was enhancement in the treated site on postgadolinium MRI scans despite normal posttreatment angiograms.[90]

No ideal embolic material has been identified for preradiotherapy use. Most centers, however, recommend the use of more permanent agents, such as cyanoacrylate polymers or Onyx, which is an ethylene vinyl alcohol copolymer dissolved in dimethyl sulfoxide (DMSO), because of several reports that less durable agents may result in approximately 16% recanalization rates after radiosurgery.[91] There is also some evidence, however, that the use of newer, more permanent agents may result in a recanalization rate of 11.8%.[88] The late recanalization may be dependent on the concentration of acrylic deposited within the nidus.[88,92,93] Flow reduction alone without evidence of reduction of AVM volume may not provide any benefit before radiotherapy and may make it more difficult to determine a conformal dose plan at the time of radiotherapy planning.[91]

Targeted Therapy

Target embolization can be performed to occlude high-risk lesions, such as intranidal or flow-related aneurysms before surgical or radiosurgical treatments (**Fig. 2**). Similarly, in some patients with high-grade AVMs not suitable for surgical resection or curative endovascular embolization, partial treatment targeted to eliminate an identified bleeding source is undertaken.

Aneurysms are often identified in association with AVMs and represent an additional source of potential morbidity that must be considered in formulating treatment of AVM patients.[47,94,95] Both intra- and extranidal aneurysms are considered risk factors for ICH in patients with AVMs.[94,96] Redekop and colleagues noted ICH associated with 38% of their series of 632 AVMs. Presentation with ICH occurred in 72% of patients with intranidal aneurysms; 36% without aneurysms; and 40% with flow-related or unrelated aneurysms. The investigators also found an annual hemorrhage rate of nearly 10% among patients with intranidal aneurysms who were not treated.[51] Hence, endovascular treatment should be targeted to close the feeding pedicle from which the aneurysm originates first to minimize the chance of subsequent hemorrhage. Alternatively, intranidal aneurysms may be addressed by surgical resection of the entire AVM.

Differing recommendations have been made for the treatment of feeding artery aneurysms in conjunction with AVM hemorrhage. Thompson and colleagues[97] found that of 45 aneurysms identified in 600 patients, five bled before treatment whereas two bled within 3 weeks after AVM treatment. Their experience and others[98] led to the recommendation that aneurysms on feeding arteries should be treated before definitive treatment of the AVM. Other investigators suggest, however, that decreasing flow through the AVM results in frequent regression of extranidal aneurysms without the need for direct treatment. For example, one study reported complete spontaneous regression of aneurysm on distal feeding arteries in 80% of cases after curative therapy of the AVM.[51] Meisel and colleagues[99] also reported significant regression of feeding artery aneurysms after treatment of the AVM. In 83 treated patients with 149 proximally located aneurysms, they found complete regression in 8% and more than 50% shrinkage in 22%. The shrinkage of proximally located aneurysms was influenced by the degree of AVM occlusion and occurred faster for those aneurysms on midline vessels, such as the anterior cerebral artery and circle of Willis. Thus, proximally located flow-related aneurysms should not be

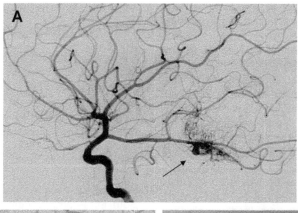

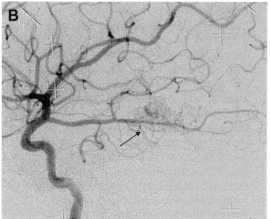
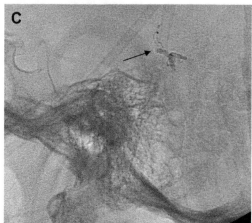

Fig. 2. Treatment of distal feeding artery aneurysm of the posterior cerebral artery in a patient with ruptured AVM before (*A*) and after (*B*) NBCA embolization. (*C*) The NBCA cast. *Dark arrow* represents distal feeding artery aneurysm (*A*). *Dark arrow* represents complete obliteration of distal feeding artery aneurysm (*B*).

prioritized in cases where the AVM is the source of hemorrhage. If the feeding artery is identified as the case of an acute hemorrhage, it should be treated as any ruptured aneurysm.

Curative Embolization

AVMs can also be cured completely using embolization alone (**Fig. 3**). Published embolization cure rates range from 9.7% to 14%.[6,88,100,101] The numbers vary, however, depending on selection criteria and technique.

The chance of a cure rate seems inversely proportional to the AVM volume and the number of feeding pedicles. Wikholm and colleagues[6] reported success as heavily dependent on the size of the AVM nidus with complete obliteration rates of 71% with AVMs smaller than 4 mL and only 15% with AVMs ranging from 4 to 8 mL. Conversely, Valavanis et al did not find that AVM volume significantly predicted the potential for endovascular cure. Rather, they had a 74% rate of curative embolization in a subgroup of patients with favorable angiographic features, such as one or few dominant feeding arteries, no perinidal angiogenesis, and a fistulous nidus.[102] Overall, these authors reported a 40% cure rate in a series of 387 consecutive patients.[102]

With improved techniques and growing experience, the proportions of AVMs that are successfully obliterated with embolizations are increasing. The introduction of Onyx as an embolic material for AVMs a few years ago has made embolization more successful in obliterating larger parts of the AVM and has resulted in complete obliteration rates as high as 18% to 49%.[103–106] The reason for this success lies in the nature of the material itself, which allows for prolonged and repeated injections, resulting in deeper penetration into the AVM nidus. The material also allows the procedure to be performed more safely due to better control of embolic material distribution.

Palliative Embolization

Palliative embolization does not seem to improve on conservative medical management of patients with incurable AVMs and may even worsen the

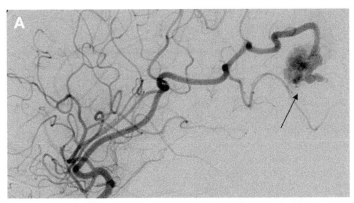

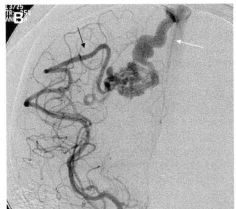
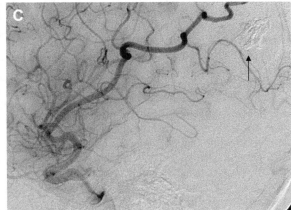

Fig. 3. Curative AVM embolization. (*A*) Lateral angiogram shows parieto-occipital AVM nidus (*arrow*). (*B*) Antero-posterior view shows single feeding artery (*dark arrow*) and superficial draining vein (*white arrow*). (*C*) Lateral postembolization angiogram shows complete obliteration of the nidus.

subsequent clinical course.[107] There is evidence that indicates that partial treatment of large AVMs—with embolization or surgery—increases the risk of subsequent ICH.[4–6]

There is, however, a role for palliative embolization in select circumstances. It can alleviate symptoms due to arterial steal or secondary to venous hypertension. It is often only temporary, however, because collaterals develop rapidly, reducing the effectiveness of the therapy. It may also be undertaken in patients presenting with seizures resistant to medical management. It is believed that partial embolization reduces the severity of arterial shunting and thereby improves perfusion pressure in the surrounding functional brain parenchyma. Evidence for this strategy comes from a few small series.[49,108] Another study reported improvement in motor weakness after palliative embolization of large AVMs located in the rolandic motor cortex.[109]

NEUROENDOVASCULAR PROCEDURE

Access for the embolization procedure is achieved through the femoral artery with placement of a 5- or 6-French sheath. Anticoagulation decisions for AVMs are made on a case-by-case basis. Some centers prefer to use heparin to keep the ACT greater than 2 to 2.5 the baseline; other centers do not use heparin. Typically, a 5 or 6 French guiding catheter and a flow-directed microcatheter are used for the embolization procedure. The guiding catheter is attached to continuous heparinized saline flush via a pressurized bag.

Most centers perform embolizations under general anesthesia, and some use neuroelectrophysiologic monitoring (somatosensory evoked potentials and electroencephalography) to monitor neurologic function during the procedure. Others use monitored anesthesia care with deep intravenous sedation. There is no evidence that general endotracheal anesthesia or monitored anesthesia care is associated with a lower rate of complications.[110] Both methods have advantages and disadvantages. Arguments for embolization under general anesthesia include improved visualization of structures with the absence of patient movement, especially with temporary apnea or when the ventilator is correlated with digital subtraction angiography contrast injection. Hypotension may be induced to slow the flow through the fistula and provide a more controlled deposition of embolic material, particularly if NBCA is being used.

Monitored anesthesia care trades off the potential for patient movement for increased knowledge of the true functional anatomy of a given patient. This approach demands deep intravenous sedation, however, to render patients comfortable during catheter placement yet keep patients appropriately responsive for selective neurologic testing. In this setting, superselective injection of amobarbital (Amytal) with or without lidocaine into the feeder vessel is performed before AVM embolization.[111–113] Focused neurologic examination is then immediately performed. The evoked deficits resolve with dissipation of the injected agent within several minutes.

Rauch and colleagues reported their experience with 147 embolizations of supratentorial AVMs after Amytal tests in 30 awake patients.[111–113] Two out of five embolizations performed after a positive Amytal test were followed by neurologic complications. Conversely, none of the 82 embolizations performed as single embolizations immediately after a negative Amytal test were associated with neurologic complications. The investigators highlighted the importance of concomitant EEG evaluation because many patients develop EEG changes in the absence of clinical symptoms.

EMBOLIC AGENTS

There are many different embolic agents currently available: liquid embolysates (NBCA, Onyx, and ethanol [ETOH] particles (PVA particles), and solid

occlusive devices (coils, silk, threads, and balloons).

Liquid Embolysates

Liquid embolysates are the most widely used and most effective agents for AVM embolization. The two most commonly used are the cyanoacrylate polymers (eg, NBCA, Trufill, Cordis Endovascular, Warren, NJ), often referred to as glue, and Onyx (ev3 Inc, Irvine, CA)-an ethylene vinyl alcohol copolymer dissolved in dimethyl sulfoxide (**Fig. 4**). In contrast to NBCA, Onyx is a liquid nonadhesive and cohesive embolic agent that was only approved by the US Food and Drug Administration (FDA) in July 2005. Finally, ETOH, which has been used effectively to treat peripheral AVMs, has also been applied with some success for the treatment of central nervous system lesions.[114]

Liquid adhesive polymer agents offer several important advantages: (1) the potential for penetration deep into the AVM nidus; (2) permanent embolization with durable obliteration of the vessel or pedicle; (3) the ability to be delivered through small, flexible, flow-directed catheters that can be manipulated safely and atraumatically into the most distal locations within the cerebrovasculature; and (4) the ability to be delivered into the pedicle quickly.

n-butyl-cyanoacrylate
NBCA was approved by the FDA for presurgical embolization of cerebral vascular malformations in 2000. NBCA is a liquid monomer that undergoes a rapid exothermic polymerization catalyzed by

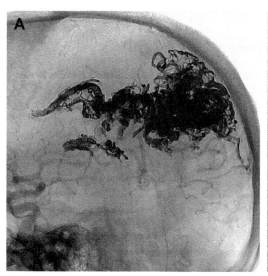 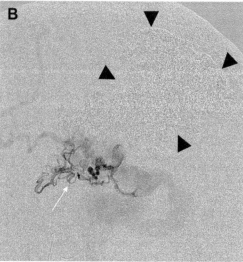

Fig. 4. (*A*) Demonstrates a large Onyx cast of a ruptured right parietal AVM. (*B*) The extent of Onyx embolization is marked with small dark arrowheads. The remaining nidus was treated with Onyx from microcatheter position shown by white arrow. The anterior circulation supply was nearly completely eliminated by embolization. An area posterior to the inferiormost cast (not shown) was treated with radiosurgery.

nucleophiles found in blood and on the vascular endothelium to form an adhesive solid. The rate of polymerization can be adjusted by mixing ethiodized oil into the mixture, which, unlike NBCA, is also radio-opaque. Higher concentrations of ethiodized oil decrease the polymerization rate and increase the viscosity of the embolic material. Ratios used in a prospective, randomized clinical study of the NBCA liquid embolic system varied from 10% to 70% NBCA and 30% to 80% ethiodized oil by volume. Typically, a 1:1 to 1:3 (NBCA:oil) mixture is used for most embolizations. This translates into 2 to 7 seconds polymerization time. Modifications can be made based on an individual's angioarchitecture and hemodynamics. Glacial acetic acid may be added in low concentrations to delay polymerization and lead to increased penetration. This technique is, however, a deviation from the FDA-approved indications for use of the commercially available NBCA. Tantalum powder may be mixed with the NBCA:oil mixture to provide greater radio-opacity. The goal of the embolization is to form a solid intranidal NBCA cast, avoiding early polymerization in the arterial feeder or later polymerization in the venous outflow. Pure NBCA polymerizes almost instantaneously at the catheter tip.

NBCA is a permanent embolic agent. The vessel is permanently occluded when the polymer completely fills the lumen. NBCA provokes an inflammatory response in the wall of the vessel and surrounding tissue, leading to vessel necrosis and fibrous ingrowth.[6] Although recanalization can occur, it is uncommon after an adequate embolization.

N-butyl-cyanoacrylate technique Pedicles targeted for embolization are identified on the initial angiographic images. The microcatheter is navigated primarily using a flow-directed technique. The microwire is generally maintained within the confines of the catheter, functioning to add support to the proximal aspects of the catheter as it is advanced distally. After the microcatheter has been successfully manipulated into a perinidal position, a gentle injection of contrast is performed on a blank roadmap. If the fluoroscopic images demonstrate catheterization of a potential pedicle for embolization, a superselective digital subtraction angiographic image is acquired. A higher frame rate is sometimes helpful, particularly if the pedicle courses into a region with brisk arteriovenous shunting to identify contrast opacification distinctly in various stages.

The image acquired from microcatheter injection is then reviewed. Four primary considerations when evaluating the superselective injection images are as follows: (1) the identification of any normal parenchymal branches arising from the pedicle to be embolized; with a few exceptions, pedicles that give rise to viable parenchymal branches should not be embolized; (2) the anatomy of the catheterized pedicle proximal to the catheter tip and AVM nidus—specifically, the identification of, localization of, and origin of any eloquent branches arising from the targeted pedicle that could be compromised by reflux; (3) the rate of transit of contrast through the nidus; if brisk arteriovenous shunting is present, it may be helpful to reduce the systolic blood pressure to 90 mm Hg or lower during embolization; and (4) the anatomy and transit time of the draining vein that appears first.[72]

The positioning of the microcatheter in terms of the orientation of the pedicle and the location of the nidus are critical. A view should be chosen that elongates the microcatheter and proximally should not overlap with the nidus or the draining vein. This orientation facilitates the early visualization of reflux, thus minimizing the risk of gluing the catheter in place or occluding proximal eloquent branches. This is also relevant for occlusion of a draining vein.

After the microcatheter is purged with a solution of 5% dextrose in water, the NBCA injection is performed with the patient apneic under blank fluoroscopic roadmap control for patients under general anesthesia. When the desired NBCA cast is achieved, the microcatheter is gently aspirated and briskly removed from the patient. A control angiogram is then obtained to evaluate the status of the nidus, the draining veins, and any complications that may have occurred. Special attention is given to evaluate for any evidence of contrast extravasation, indicating bleeding.

Ethylene-vinyl alcohol copolymer with dimethyl sulfoxide

Onyx is a nonadhesive liquid embolic agent with a lava-like flow pattern. It is premixed with EVOH, DMSO, and micronized tantalum powder for radio-opacity. EVOH contains 48 mol/L ethylene and 53 mol/L vinyl alcohol.[115] The copolymer holds together as it is injected but it does not adhere to the endothelium or to the microcatheter tip. When the mixture contacts aqueous media, such as blood, DMSO rapidly diffuses away from the mixture, causing in situ precipitation and solidification of the polymer, with formation of a spongy embolus. This solidification occurs more slowly than that of cyanoacrylates, and, because Onyx is nonadherent to the walls of the vessel or microcatheter, this material allows prolonged injection times while decreasing the chances of permanent microcatheter retention. The precipitation progresses from the outer surface inward, forming a skin with a liquid center that continues to flow as the solidification continues. The rate of precipitation of the copolymer is proportional to the concentration of EVOH.

DMSO has adverse effects. It can induce vasospasm, angionecrosis, arterial thrombosis, and vascular rupture.[116,117] These undesirable consequences are related to the volume of DMSO infused and the endothelial contact time. Severe angiotoxic effects do not occur when the DMSO infusion rate does not exceed 0.25 mL/90 s.[118] Only specifically approved microcatheters (Ultraflow, Marathon, and Echelon; ev3) can be used with Onyx because the DMSO dissolves incompatible catheters. Patients may notice a garlic-like taste for several hours, and their skin and breath may have a characteristic odor due to the DMSO for 1 to 2 days after an embolization with Onyx.

Onyx intended for use in AVM embolization is manufactured as Onyx 18 (6% EVOH) and Onyx 34 (8% EVOH). Generally, Onyx 18 is used for embolization of a plexiform nidus, and Onyx 34 is used for embolization of large arteriovenous shunts in the AVM. Onyx 18 travels further distally and penetrates more deeply into the nidus because of its lower viscosity and slower precipitation rate. Complete solidification of both formulations occurs within 5 minutes. Before injection, Onyx solution must be vigorously shaken for 20 minutes to fully suspend the micronized tantalum powder. The manufacturer provides an adapted Vortex-Genie (Scientific Industries, Bohemia, New York) to mix the Onyx. Mixing is continued until just before the embolization. Failure to do so may result in inadequate radio-opacity.[115]

Due to its properties and increased predictability, the use of Onyx may allow for more controlled injections with better distal nidus or fistula penetration when compared with cyanoacrylate. In addition, control angiography can be performed during the embolization to assess the status of the AVM nidus and draining veins and to rule out nontarget embolization. Fluoroscopy times are typically longer than with the use of cyanoacrylate, however.

Onyx technique Once an Onyx-compatible microcatheter is positioned in the desired location using flow-directed and guide wire–assisted navigation, a superselective angiogram is obtained. This is followed by a guide-catheter angiography using the same projection and magnification. Reference images of the microcatheter and of the guide catheter angiograms on the early arterial, parenchymal, and late venous phases are saved. These reference images can be quickly flipped back and forth during the Onyx injection and can be extremely helpful in answering questions about where the embolic agent is flowing.

The technique and pace of an Onyx injection is distinct from NBCA and is termed the "plug-and-push technique." Reflux is promoted during the initial phases of the injection to allow forming a solid plug at the microcatheter tip and subsequently promote anterograde flow. Forming an early dense reflux plug allows greater nidal depositions while ultimately minimizing the amount of reflux. The rationale for this technique is counterintuitive but relatively simple. The older the Onyx deposition is, the more solid the embolus, thereby forcing subsequent Onyx to deposit anterograde. Conversely, prioritizing anterograde deposition makes it harder for subsequent Onyx to break through, and develops more reflux.

An early proximal plug can be more easily built with the initial use of Onyx 34 for two reasons: (1) the higher concentration of the EVOH copolymer in Onyx 34 increases its viscosity, which makes a proximal deposition/early reflux more likely, and (2) the lower concentration of DMSO in Onyx 34 leads to a faster precipitation and consequently to a denser early plug.

At the beginning of the embolization procedure, the microcatheter is flushed with 5 mL of saline. DMSO and Onyx 34 are prepared in two different 1-mL syringes. The dead space of the microcatheter is then slowly filled with DMSO and the microcatheter hub is bathed with DMSO forming a meniscus.

Onyx is slowly injected over 90 seconds to fill the microcatheter and replace the DMSO in the dead space. Fast injections of DMSO may result in vasospasm or even angionecrosis. The goal of this initial injection is to stay as proximal to the microcatheter as possible; therefore, the injection is halted if any antegrade deposition is observed. A waiting time of 30 to 90 seconds is typically allowed in this case. Pauses longer than 2 minutes may result in Onyx solidification within the microcatheter. The initial objective is to form a dense Onyx cast around the tip of the microcatheter and with reflux over a short distance (5–7 mm) with only minimal initial antegrade deposition. After a dense retrograde plug is formed, the antegrade Onyx injection is started with 1 mL of Onyx 34 and then switched to Onyx 18 for the remainder of the embolization procedure. The process of breaking through this early plug may result in additional initial reflux and several injection pauses may be required before an antegrade deposition occurs. Careful observation of the blank roadmap and native fluoroscopic images is essential during this phase of nidal deposition, preferably using biplane technology and with the assistance of a second operator who should focus in the appearance of new reflux. Injection pauses of 30 to 120 seconds are performed whenever unwanted reflux or flow into nontarget areas (eg, different arterial pedicles or venous outflow region) is observed. This seems to allow for precipitation of the Onyx at those areas, which results in diversion of the newly injected Onyx to other areas. Using this technique it is not uncommon that large volumes of Onyx are injected into the AVM nidus from one single microcatheter position. Typically, only one to two pedicles per session are injected.

The injection should be terminated under the following circumstances: (1) the targeted portion of the nidus has been embolized; (2) concerns about venous outflow obstruction or slowing of venous flow arise; (3) excess of reflux; or (4) resistance to injection increases significantly as this may precede rupture of the microcatheter or vessel. The amount of tolerated reflux varies depending on several factors, including (1) the existence of proximal branches; (2) the caliber of the vessel embolized; (3) the tortuousity of the proximal vessels; and (4) the density of the existent reflux. After the injection is completed, the syringe is aspirated gently and gentle traction is gradually applied to remove the microcatheter. There is a broad variation in the amount of time required for microcatheter removal depending on the length and density of the reflux and the proximal tortuousity and caliber of the vessels embolized. Retrieval times up to 90 minutes have been observed.[119] As in every other stage of Onyx embolization, patience is essential. It is common for the Onyx cast to show some deflection while traction is applied to the microcatheter. The slow traction method, which uses incremental catheter withdrawal (centimeter by centimeter) with sustained moderate tension on the catheter, is the best method to retrieve the catheter. Constant microcatheter traction should then be maintained for a few minutes before additional traction is applied. Although stretching may promote thinning of the distal portion of the microcatheter and, therefore, facilitate its extraction, it may also translate into a higher chance of microcatheter fracture. If the microcatheter cannot be retrieved without excessive stress on the cast or vasculature, it should be left in place and cut off at its end at the groin.

Although Onyx is a promising embolic agent, only limited long-term data are currently available for Onyx. At present, Onyx is considered a permanent agent.[106,115,120] Several studies have examined the feasibility and safety of Onyx in AVM embolization. Von Rooij and colleagues[105] reported an average size reduction of 75% after Onyx embolization in 44 patients. Total obliteration was achieved in 16% of the treated patients (all of which were Spetzler-Martin grades I and II) at the cost of mortality and permanent morbidity rates of 2.3% and 4.6%, respectively. Weber and colleagues described a complete obliteration rate of 20% after Onyx embolization alone in 93 patients harboring 94 brain AVMs. Two angiographic recurrences were evident at 3 months' follow-up, resulting in a complete obliteration rate of 18%. The overall procedural complication rate was 12% (11 cases), including clinically significant deficits (modified Rankin scale >2) in five patients (5%) and acute ICH in two patients (2%).[103,106]

Mounayer and colleagues reported their experience in the treatment of 94 brain AVM patients. A total of 210 embolizations was performed, with Onyx as the sole embolic agent in 88 procedures, Onyx and NBCA in combination in 50 procedures, and NBCA alone in 72 procedures. At the time of their report, angiographic cure was accomplished in 26 of the 53 patients (49%) in whom endovascular treatment had been completed. Procedure-related permanent neurologic deficits were observed in eight (8.5%, 8/94) patients and another three (3.2%, 3/94) patients died from procedure-related complications.[104] Katsaridis and colleagues described their experience with Onyx in the curative embolization of 101 brain AVM patients. At the time of their report, treatment had been concluded in 52 of the patients. Complete AVM obliteration was obtained in 28 patients (53.9% of the completely treated and 27.7% of all patients) and near-total occlusion was obtained in another 18 patients. The rates of permanent morbidity and mortality were 8% (8/101) and 3% (3/101), respectively.[103,106]

Ethanol

Embolization of brain AVMs with undiluted absolute ETOH (98% dehydrated alcohol injection) has been advocated on the basis of its success to eradicate peripheral vascular malformations. ETOH has a direct toxic effect on the endothelium resulting in acute thrombosis of the vessel. For the embolization procedure, ETOH is mixed with a contrast medium, most commonly ethiodized oil.

To date, only one group has reported results of brain AVM embolization with ETOH in 17 patients. They were able to cure seven patients with ETOH alone (42%). Despite this impressive cure rate, two patients with partially treated lesions died and eight patients experienced complications related to therapy.[121]

If large amounts of absolute alcohol enter the systemic circulation, toxic effects can occur; therefore, ETOH (1 mg/kg) is the maximum amount that can be injected during a single session. High-dose ETOH has been found to induce pulmonary precapillary vasospasm, leading to cardiopulmonary arrest. In addition, ETOH causes significant brain edema, necessitating treatment with high doses of steroids before and 2 weeks after treatment.

Given those risks and the relative widespread experience and comfort level with cyanoacrylates and now Onyx, there has been a general reluctance among most neurointerventionalists to use ETOH for the embolization of brain AVMs.

Particles

Polyvinyl alcohol

PVA particles were commonly used for brain AVM embolization before liquid embolic agents became more widely used.[76,122,123] PVA particles are supplied by the manufacturer in different sizes ranging from 150 μm to 1000 μm. They are nonradiopaque and are mixed with iodinated contrast for delivery.

PVA particles have several disadvantages compared with embolic agents. They are radiolucent making it impossible to identify where they deposit, and they tend to occlude the small flow-directed microcatheters. Migration of particles in normal adjacent branches is more likely because catheterization is less distal than with the flexible microcatheters used with liquid embolic agents. Furthermore, different arteriovenous shunt sizes may be observed within the nidus, which carries the risk that the particles may reach the venous side in some instances and produce no embolization efficacy or, on the contrary, inadvertent venous occlusion. To avoid migration, neurointerventionalists have first placed coils into large arteriovenous shunts in an attempt to prevent particles migrating into the pulmonary circulation.

Recanalization is more frequent than with liquid embolic agents. It has been reported on the order of 12% to 43%.[124,125] This happens because particles may aggregate and occlude the arterial feeder rather than the nidus, which then can lead to recruitment of collateral supply and regrowth of the nidus.[125] In general, this lack of durable occlusion, however, may not be a significant disadvantage for preoperative embolizations with PVA particles. A prospective, randomized, multicenter trial concluded that PVA and NBCA were similar in safety and effectiveness for preoperative brain AVM embolization.[82]

Coils

There are two different types of coils that can be used for embolization, the detachable (eg, Guglielmi detachable coils) and the non-detachable coils, including pushable coils, and the injectable Berenstein Liquid Coils. They are both useful for the obliteration of large arteriovenous fistulae within the AVM nidus. The coil is selected on the basis of the size of the feeding artery as estimated on superselective angiography or guiding catheter angiography. Detachable coils can be manipulated within the feeding artery to achieve optimal positioning, and nondetachable coils can be visualized under fluoroscopy to provide some indication of its stability within the artery. After detachment, a second coil is immediately introduced, and this is repeated until a stable basket is formed. One or more liquid coils may then be deployed. Finally, after the coil pack has adequately slowed flow through the fistula, the pedicle may be occluded with injection of a liquid embolic agent.

When detachable coils are used, the over-the-wire manipulation of a microcatheter with two distal markers into the pedicle is necessary, introducing the potential for vascular perforation. The introduction of coils into friable arterial feeders of an AVM also presents a risk of perforation. Finally, if the coils are improperly sized, there is the potential for embolization through the fistula and into the venous system.

If the arterial pedicle supplying the fistula is small enough, embolization with injectable or small pushable coils can be chosen. Liquid coils may be introduced through the smaller internal diameter, flexible, flow-directed microcatheters, eliminating the need for an exclusively over-the-wire catheterization. After the introduction of the coils sufficiently slows the transit through the fistula, occlusion can be once again achieved safely with a liquid embolic agent.

COMPLICATIONS

Complications during endovascular navigation of the cerebral vasculature can be rapid and dramatic and require interdisciplinary collaboration. Embolization of brain AVMs can be performed with a high degree of technical success and a low rate of permanent neurologic complications. The reported incidence of overall complications from brain AVM embolization varies between 3% and 25%.[78,126,127] Mortality rates associated with embolization have been reported to be 2% or less, and permanent neurologic deficits 2%

to 8.9% with the use of new-generation microcatheters.[76,77,128,129]

Microcatheter Retention

There is a risk of liquid agents adhering to the catheter, making withdrawal traumatic or impossible. Retention of the microcather tip in the nidus occurs in less than 3% of all embolizations. Retained catheters can be removed with AVM surgical resection soon after embolization or even few weeks after if there is no adhesion to the vessel wall. Straight microcatheters within the vessel lumen do not seem to cause thrombosis. Some neurointerventionalists prefer a 3- to 6-months' course of anticoagulation, however, to prevent thrombosis if deemed safe for patients.[130] Microcatheter fracture/retention may be more frequent in Onyx embolzations compared with NBCA.

Ischemic Complications

Catheter-induced thromboemboli, nontarget embolization and reflux of embolic material into normal cerebral vessels are the most common causes of cerebral ischemia during AVM embolization. Thrombotic emboli can be prevented with systemic heparinization or flush of all catheters with heparinized saline. Reflux of embolic material into normal parenchymal branches during embolization can be prevented with high-quality imaging systems, general anesthesia, optimal positioning of the microcatheter, and appropriate dilution of the liquid embolic agent to allow for desired polymerization times.[130]

Intracranial Hemorrhage

ICH, during or after embolization, represents one of the most feared complications of AVM treatment. In the setting of a hemorrhagic complication during the procedure, immediate protamine reversal of heparin (if heparin was used during the procedure) should be done as rapidly as possible.[131]

Hemorrhagic complication rates associated with embolization range from 2% to 4.7%. The possible causes are diverse but most frequently include (1) vessel perforation during microcatheter navigation (however, the use of flow-directed catheters has significantly reduced the incidence of vessel perforations as they do not require metal guide wires beyond the tip to navigate into the AVM feeders);[130] (2) venous outflow obstruction related to venous occlusion by the embolic material or late venous thrombosis due to abrupt venous flow reduction; and (3) normal perfusion pressure breakthrough (NPPB) hemorrhage.

NPPB is thought to be secondary to the sudden increase in perfusion pressure in the surrounding normal brain parenchyma, which suffers from chronically impaired autoregulation, after AVM embolization or resection. NPPB tends to occur in patients with large high-flow AVMs and multiple large feeding vessels. Reduction of a patient's mean arterial pressure 15% to 20% below the baseline during the first 24 hours after embolization and limiting embolization to 30% of the AVM nidus per session are strategies to reduce the risk of ICH due to NPPB.

Intraventricular hemorrhage may cause hydrocephalus. Hydrocephalus may require insertion of ventricular drainage catheters, which can also be used to monitor intracranial pressure. Compression of the aqueduct of Sylvius by large draining veins can also result in hydrocephalus.[73] Finally, choroidal AVMs may be associated with overproduction of CSF and hydrocephalus.

POSTPROCEDURAL CARE

Recommendations for postprocedural care include neurologic intensive care monitoring for at least 24 hours. The arterial sheath is usually removed after the procedure. Patients are preferably extubated after the procedure to allow for neurologic examinations to monitor patient condition.

Postprocedural heparinization should be considered for patients with sluggish venous outflow or compromise of an important component of the venous outflow system. Sluggish flow in the veins can lead to venous thrombosis with subsequent hemorrhage from the remaining nidus. In general, a low systolic blood pressure (100–140 mm Hg) is maintained after embolization procedures to avoid the theoretic possibility of NPPB hemorrhage. A nicardipine or labetalol drip is the preferred IV antihypertensive medication.

A new neurologic deficit after embolization is usually investigated with a CT scan to rule out a new ICH or hydrocephalus. MRI scanning with diffusion-weighted imaging may be appropriate if an ischemic infarct is under consideration or in cases where a large Onyx cast may prevent adequate CT evaluation.

REFERENCES

1. Stapf C, Mast H, Sciacca RR, et al. The New York Islands AVM Study: design, study progress, and initial results. Stroke 2003;34:e29–33.
2. Mohr JP. Stroke: pathophysiology, diagnosis, and management. 4th edition. Philadelphia: Churchill Livingstone; 2004.

3. Rinkel GJ. Intracranial aneurysm screening: indications and advice for practice. Lancet Neurol 2005; 4:122–8.

4. Han PP, Ponce FA, Spetzler RF. Intention-to-treat analysis of Spetzler-Martin grades IV and V arteriovenous malformations: natural history and treatment paradigm. J Neurosurg 2003;98:3–7.

5. Miyamoto S, Hashimoto N, Nagata I, et al. Post-treatment sequelae of palliatively treated cerebral arteriovenous malformations. Neurosurgery 2000; 46:589–94.

6. Wikholm G, Lundqvist C, Svendsen P. Embolization of cerebral arteriovenous malformations: part I–technique, morphology, and complications. Neurosurgery 1996;39:448–57.

7. Perret G, Nishioka H. Report on the cooperative study of intracranial aneurysms and subarachnoid hemorrhage. Section VI. Arteriovenous malformations. An analysis of 545 cases of cranio-cerebral arteriovenous malformations and fistulae reported to the cooperative study. J Neurosurg 1966;25: 467–90.

8. McCormick WF, Rosenfield DB. Massive brain hemorrhage: a review of 144 cases and an examination of their causes. Stroke 1973;4:946–54.

9. Jessurun GA, Kamphuis DJ, van der Zande FH, et al. Cerebral arteriovenous malformations in The Netherlands Antilles. High prevalence of hereditary hemorrhagic telangiectasia-related single and multiple cerebral arteriovenous malformations. Clin Neurol Neurosurg 1993;95:193–8.

10. Brown RD Jr, Wiebers DO, Torner JC, et al. Frequency of intracranial hemorrhage as a presenting symptom and subtype analysis: a population-based study of intracranial vascular malformations in Olmsted Country, Minnesota. J Neurosurg 1996; 85:29–32.

11. Brown RD Jr, Wiebers DO, Torner JC, et al. Incidence and prevalence of intracranial vascular malformations in Olmsted County, Minnesota, 1965 to 1992. Neurology 1996;46:949–52.

12. Kadoya C, Momota Y, Ikegami Y, et al. Central nervous system arteriovenous malformations with hereditary hemorrhagic telangiectasia: report of a family with three cases. Surg Neurol 1994;42:234–9.

13. Ruigrok YM, Rinkel GJ, Wijmenga C. Genetics of intracranial aneurysms. Lancet Neurol 2005;4: 179–89.

14. Willinsky RA, Lasjaunias P, Terbrugge K, et al. Multiple cerebral arteriovenous malformations (AVMs). Review of our experience from 203 patients with cerebral vascular lesions. Neuroradiology 1990;32:207–10.

15. Herzig R, Burval S, Vladyka V, et al. Familial occurrence of cerebral arteriovenous malformation in sisters: case report and review of the literature. Eur J Neurol 2000;7:95–100.

16. Chaloupka JC, Huddle DC. Classification of vascular malformations of the central nervous system. Neuroimaging Clin N Am 1998;8:295–321.

17. Mullan S, Mojtahedi S, Johnson DL, et al. Embryological basis of some aspects of cerebral vascular fistulas and malformations. J Neurosurg 1996;85: 1–8.

18. Friedman JA, Pollock BE, Nichols DA. Development of a cerebral arteriovenous malformation documented in an adult by serial angiography. Case report. J Neurosurg 2000;93:1058–61.

19. Hashimoto N, Nozaki K. Do cerebral arteriovenous malformations recur after angiographically confirmed total extirpation? Crit Rev Neurosurg 1999;9:141–6.

20. Kader A, Goodrich JT, Sonstein WJ, et al. Recurrent cerebral arteriovenous malformations after negative postoperative angiograms. J Neurosurg 1996; 85:14–8.

21. Kupersmith MJ, Vargas ME, Yashar A, et al. Occipital arteriovenous malformations: visual disturbances and presentation. Neurology 1996;46: 953–7.

22. Lobato RD, Rivas JJ, Gomez PA, et al. Comparison of the clinical presentation of symptomatic arteriovenous malformations (angiographically visualized) and occult vascular malformations. Neurosurgery 1992;31:391–6.

23. Brown RD Jr, Wiebers DO, Forbes G, et al. The natural history of unruptured intracranial arteriovenous malformations. J Neurosurg 1988;68:352–7.

24. Mast H, Mohr JP, Osipov A, et al. 'Steal' is an unestablished mechanism for the clinical presentation of cerebral arteriovenous malformations. Stroke 1995; 26:1215–20.

25. Wilkins RH. Natural history of intracranial vascular malformations: a review. Neurosurgery 1985;16: 421–30.

26. Lees F. The migrainous symptoms of cerebral angiomata. J Neurol Neurosurg Psychiatry 1962;25: 45–50.

27. Evans RW. Diagnostic testing for the evaluation of headaches. Neurol Clin 1996;14:1–26.

28. ApSimon HT, Reef H, Phadke RV, et al. A population-based study of brain arteriovenous malformation: long-term treatment outcomes. Stroke 2002; 33:2794–800.

29. Halim AX, Johnston SC, Singh V, et al. Longitudinal risk of intracranial hemorrhage in patients with arteriovenous malformation of the brain within a defined population. Stroke 2004;35:1697–702.

30. Hillman J. Population-based analysis of arteriovenous malformation treatment. J Neurosurg 2001; 95:633–7.

31. Hofmeister C, Stapf C, Hartmann A, et al. Demographic, morphological, and clinical characteristics of 1289 patients with brain arteriovenous malformation. Stroke 2000;31:1307–10.

32. Khaw AV, Mohr JP, Sciacca RR, et al. Association of infratentorial brain arteriovenous malformations with hemorrhage at initial presentation. Stroke 2004;35:660–3.

33. Miyasaka Y, Kurata A, Tanaka R, et al. Mass effect caused by clinically unruptured cerebral arteriovenous malformations. Neurosurgery 1997;41:1060–3.

34. Aminoff MJ. Treatment of unruptured cerebral arteriovenous malformations. Neurology 1987;37: 815–9.

35. Jane JA, Kassell NF, Torner JC, et al. The natural history of aneurysms and arteriovenous malformations. J Neurosurg 1985;62:321–3.

36. Ondra SL, Troupp H, George ED, et al. The natural history of symptomatic arteriovenous malformations of the brain: a 24-year follow-up assessment. J Neurosurg 1990;73:387–91.

37. Forster DM, Steiner L, Hakanson S. Arteriovenous malformations of the brain. A long-term clinical study. J Neurosurg 1972;37:562–70.

38. Graf CJ, Perret GE, Torner JC. Bleeding from cerebral arteriovenous malformations as part of their natural history. J Neurosurg 1983;58:331–7.

39. Fults D, Kelly DL Jr. Natural history of arteriovenous malformations of the brain: a clinical study. Neurosurgery 1984;15:658–62.

40. Mast H, Young WL, Koennecke HC, et al. Risk of spontaneous haemorrhage after diagnosis of cerebral arteriovenous malformation. Lancet 1997;350: 1065–8.

41. Itoyama Y, Uemura S, Ushio Y, et al. Natural course of unoperated intracranial arteriovenous malformations: study of 50 cases. J Neurosurg 1989;71:805–9.

42. Krayenbuehl H, Siebenmann R. Small vascular malformations as a cause of primary intracerebral hemorrhage. J Neurosurg 1965;22:7–20.

43. Pollock BE, Flickinger JC, Lunsford LD, et al. Factors that predict the bleeding risk of cerebral arteriovenous malformations. Stroke 1996;27:1–6.

44. Hernesniemi JA, Dashti R, Juvela S, et al. Natural history of brain arteriovenous malformations: a long-term follow-up study of risk of hemorrhage in 238 patients. Neurosurgery 2008;63:823–31.

45. Duong DH, Young WL, Vang MC, et al. Feeding artery pressure and venous drainage pattern are primary determinants of hemorrhage from cerebral arteriovenous malformations. Stroke 1998;29: 1167–76.

46. Langer DJ, Lasner TM, Hurst RW, et al. Hypertension, small size, and deep venous drainage are associated with risk of hemorrhagic presentation of cerebral arteriovenous malformations. Neurosurgery 1998;42:481–6 [discussion: 487–9].

47. Marks MP, Lane B, Steinberg GK, et al. Hemorrhage in intracerebral arteriovenous malformations: angiographic determinants. Radiology 1990;176: 807–13.

48. Miyasaka Y, Yada K, Ohwada T, et al. An analysis of the venous drainage system as a factor in hemorrhage from arteriovenous malformations. J Neurosurg 1992;76:239–43.

49. Kusske JA, Kelly WA. Embolization and reduction of the "steal" syndrome in cerebral arteriovenous malformations. J Neurosurg 1974;40:313–21.

50. Young WL, Prohovnik I, Ornstein E, et al. The effect of arteriovenous malformation resection on cerebrovascular reactivity to carbon dioxide. Neurosurgery 1990;27:257–66.

51. Redekop G, TerBrugge K, Montanera W, et al. Arterial aneurysms associated with cerebral arteriovenous malformations: classification, incidence, and risk of hemorrhage. J Neurosurg 1998;89:539–46.

52. Turjman F, Massoud TF, Vinuela F, et al. Correlation of the angioarchitectural features of cerebral arteriovenous malformations with clinical presentation of hemorrhage. Neurosurgery 1995;37:856–60.

53. Stapf C, Mast H, Sciacca RR, et al. Predictors of hemorrhage in patients with untreated brain arteriovenous malformation. Neurology 2006;66:1350–5.

54. Hartmann A, Mast H, Mohr JP, et al. Morbidity of intracranial hemorrhage in patients with cerebral arteriovenous malformation. Stroke 1998;29:931–4.

55. Laakso A, Dashti R, Seppanen J, et al. Long-term excess mortality in 623 patients with brain arteriovenous malformations. Neurosurgery 2008;63:244–53.

56. Spetzler RF, Martin NA. A proposed grading system for arteriovenous malformations. J Neurosurg 1986;65:476–83.

57. Brown RD Jr. Simple risk predictions for arteriovenous malformation hemorrhage [comment]. Neurosurgery 2000;46:1024.

58. Pertuiset B, Ancri D, Kinuta Y, et al. Classification of supratentorial arteriovenous malformations. A score system for evaluation of operability and surgical strategy based on an analysis of 66 cases. Acta Neurochir (Wien) 1991;110:6–16.

59. Shi YQ, Chen XC. A proposed scheme for grading intracranial arteriovenous malformations. J Neurosurg 1986;65:484–9.

60. Tamaki N, Ehara K, Lin TK, et al. Cerebral arteriovenous malformations: factors influencing the surgical difficulty and outcome. Neurosurgery 1991;29:856–61.

61. Hamilton MG, Spetzler RF. The prospective application of a grading system for arteriovenous malformations. Neurosurgery 1994;34:2–6.

62. Heros RC, Korosue K, Diebold PM. Surgical excision of cerebral arteriovenous malformations: late results. Neurosurgery 1990;26:570–7.

63. Lawton MT. Spetzler-Martin Grade III arteriovenous malformations: surgical results and a modification of the grading scale. Neurosurgery 2003;52:740–8.

64. Spetzler RF, Hargraves RW, McCormick PW, et al. Relationship of perfusion pressure and size to risk

of hemorrhage from arteriovenous malformations. J Neurosurg 1992;76:918–23.

65. Latchaw RE, Hu X, Ugurbil K, et al. Functional magnetic resonance imaging as a management tool for cerebral arteriovenous malformations. Neurosurgery 1995;37:619–25.

66. Schlosser MJ, McCarthy G, Fulbright RK, et al. Cerebral vascular malformations adjacent to sensorimotor and visual cortex. Functional magnetic resonance imaging studies before and after therapeutic intervention. Stroke 1997;28:1130–7.

67. Turjman F, Massoud TF, Vinuela F, et al. Aneurysms related to cerebral arteriovenous malformations: superselective angiographic assessment in 58 patients. AJNR Am J Neuroradiol 1994;15:1601–5.

68. Morris P. Practical neuroangiography. 2nd edition. Philadelphia: Lippincott Williams & Wilkins; 2007.

69. Pile-Spellman JM, Baker KF, Liszczak TM, et al. High-flow angiopathy: cerebral blood vessel changes in experimental chronic arteriovenous fistula. AJNR Am J Neuroradiol 1986;7:811–5.

70. Marks MP, Lane B, Steinberg GK, et al. Intranidal aneurysms in cerebral arteriovenous malformations: evaluation and endovascular treatment. Radiology 1992;183:355–60.

71. Valavanis A. The role of angiography in the evaluation of cerebral vascular malformations. Neuroimaging Clin N Am 1996;6:679–704.

72. Fiorella D, Albuquerque FC, Woo HH, et al. The role of neuroendovascular therapy for the treatment of brain arteriovenous malformations. Neurosurgery 2006;59:S163–77.

73. Ogilvy CS, Stieg PE, Awad I, et al. Recommendations for the management of intracranial arteriovenous malformations: a statement for healthcare professionals from a special writing group of the Stroke Council, American Stroke Association. Circulation 2001;103:2644–57.

74. Martin NA, Khanna R, Doberstein C, et al. Therapeutic embolization of arteriovenous malformations: the case for and against. Clin Neurosurg 2000;46:295–318.

75. Jafar JJ, Davis AJ, Berenstein A, et al. The effect of embolization with N-butyl cyanoacrylate prior to surgical resection of cerebral arteriovenous malformations. J Neurosurg 1993;78:60–9.

76. Purdy PD, Batjer HH, Risser RC, et al. Arteriovenous malformations of the brain: choosing embolic materials to enhance safety and ease of excision. J Neurosurg 1992;77:217–22.

77. Purdy PD, Batjer HH, Samson D, et al. Intraarterial sodium amytal administration to guide preoperative embolization of cerebral arteriovenous malformations. J Neurosurg Anesthesiol 1991;3:103–6.

78. Vinuela F, Dion JE, Duckwiler G, et al. Combined endovascular embolization and surgery in the management of cerebral arteriovenous malformations: experience with 101 cases. J Neurosurg 1991;75:856–64.

79. Morgan MK, Zurin AA, Harrington T, et al. Changing role for preoperative embolisation in the management of arteriovenous malformations of the brain. J Clin Neurosci 2000;7:527–30.

80. Hartmann A, Mast H, Mohr JP, et al. Determinants of staged endovascular and surgical treatment outcome of brain arteriovenous malformations. Stroke 2005;36:2431–5.

81. DeMeritt JS, Pile-Spellman J, Mast H, et al. Outcome analysis of preoperative embolization with N-butyl cyanoacrylate in cerebral arteriovenous malformations. AJNR Am J Neuroradiol 1995;16:1801–7.

82. N-butyl cyanoacrylate embolization of cerebral arteriovenous malformations: results of a prospective, randomized, multi-center trial. AJNR Am J Neuroradiol 2002;23:748–55.

83. Kwon Y, Jeon SR, Kim JH, et al. Analysis of the causes of treatment failure in gamma knife radiosurgery for intracranial arteriovenous malformations. J Neurosurg 2000;93(Suppl 3):104–6.

84. Lunsford LD, Kondziolka D, Flickinger JC, et al. Stereotactic radiosurgery for arteriovenous malformations of the brain. J Neurosurg 1991;75:512–24.

85. Steiner L, Lindquist C, Adler JR, et al. Clinical outcome of radiosurgery for cerebral arteriovenous malformations. J Neurosurg 1992;77:1–8.

86. Maruyama K, Kawahara N, Shin M, et al. The risk of hemorrhage after radiosurgery for cerebral arteriovenous malformations. N Engl J Med 2005;352:146–53.

87. Pollock BE. Stereotactic radiosurgery for arteriovenous malformations. Neurosurg Clin N Am 1999;10:281–90.

88. Gobin YP, Laurent A, Merienne L, et al. Treatment of brain arteriovenous malformations by embolization and radiosurgery. J Neurosurg 1996;85:19–28.

89. Henkes H, Nahser HC, Berg-Dammer E, et al. Endovascular therapy of brain AVMs prior to radiosurgery. Neurol Res 1998;20:479–92.

90. Shin M, Kawahara N, Maruyama K, et al. Risk of hemorrhage from an arteriovenous malformation confirmed to have been obliterated on angiography after stereotactic radiosurgery. J Neurosurg 2005;102:842–6.

91. Pollock BE, Kondziolka D, Lunsford LD, et al. Repeat stereotactic radiosurgery of arteriovenous malformations: factors associated with incomplete obliteration. Neurosurgery 1996;38:318–24.

92. Fournier D, Terbrugge K, Rodesch G, et al. Revascularization of brain arteriovenous malformations after embolization with bucrylate. Neuroradiology 1990;32:497–501.

93. Rao VR, Mandalam KR, Gupta AK, et al. Dissolution of isobutyl 2-cyanoacrylate on long-term follow-up. AJNR Am J Neuroradiol 1989;10:135–41.

94. Kim EJ, Halim AX, Dowd CF, et al. The relationship of coexisting extranidal aneurysms to intracranial hemorrhage in patients harboring brain arteriovenous malformations. Neurosurgery 2004;54:1349–57.

95. Lasjaunias P, Piske R, Terbrugge K, et al. Cerebral arteriovenous malformations (C. AVM) and associated arterial aneurysms (AA). Analysis of 101 C. AVM cases, with 37 AA in 23 patients. Acta Neurochir (Wien) 1988;91:29–36.

96. Brown RD Jr, Wiebers DO, Forbes GS. Unruptured intracranial aneurysms and arteriovenous malformations: frequency of intracranial hemorrhage and relationship of lesions. J Neurosurg 1990;73:859–63.

97. Thompson RC, Steinberg GK, Levy RP, et al. The management of patients with arteriovenous malformations and associated intracranial aneurysms. Neurosurgery 1998;43:202–11.

98. Ezura M, Takahashi A, Jokura H, et al. Endovascular treatment of aneurysms associated with cerebral arteriovenous malformations: experiences after the introduction of Guglielmi detachable coils. J Clin Neurosci 2000;7(Suppl 1):14–8.

99. Meisel HJ, Mansmann U, Alvarez H, et al. Cerebral arteriovenous malformations and associated aneurysms: analysis of 305 cases from a series of 662 patients. Neurosurgery 2000;46:793–800.

100. Fournier D, TerBrugge KG, Willinsky R, et al. Endovascular treatment of intracerebral arteriovenous malformations: experience in 49 cases. J Neurosurg 1991;75:228–33.

101. Vinuela F, Duckwiler G, Guglielmi G. Contribution of interventional neuroradiology in the therapeutic management of brain arteriovenous malformations. J Stroke Cerebrovasc Dis 1997;6:268–71.

102. Valavanis A, Yasargil MG. The endovascular treatment of brain arteriovenous malformations. Adv Tech Stand Neurosurg 1998;24:131–214.

103. Katsaridis V, Papagiannaki C, Aimar E. Curative embolization of cerebral arteriovenous malformations (AVMs) with Onyx in 101 patients. Neuroradiology 2008;50:589–97.

104. Mounayer C, Hammami N, Piotin M, et al. Nidal embolization of brain arteriovenous malformations using Onyx in 94 patients. AJNR Am J Neuroradiol 2007;28:518–23.

105. van Rooij WJ, Sluzewski M, Beute GN. Brain AVM embolization with Onyx. AJNR Am J Neuroradiol 2007;28:172–7.

106. Weber W, Kis B, Siekmann R, et al. Preoperative embolization of intracranial arteriovenous malformations with Onyx. Neurosurgery 2007;61:244–52.

107. Kwon OK, Han DH, Han MH, et al. Palliatively treated cerebral arteriovenous malformations: follow-up results. J Clin Neurosci 2000;7(Suppl 1):69–72.

108. Luessenhop AJ, Mujica PH. Embolization of segments of the circle of Willis and adjacent branches for management of certain inoperable cerebral arteriovenous malformations. J Neurosurg 1981;54:573–82.

109. Fox AJ, Girvin JP, Vinuela F, et al. Rolandic arteriovenous malformations: improvement in limb function by IBC embolization. AJNR Am J Neuroradiol 1985;6:575–82.

110. Manninen PH, Gignac EM, Gelb AW, et al. Anesthesia for interventional neuroradiology. J Clin Anesth 1995;7:448–52.

111. Han MH, Chang KH, Han DH, et al. Preembolization functional evaluation in supratentorial cerebral arteriovenous malformations with superselective intraarterial injection of thiopental sodium solution. Acta Radiol 1994;35:212–6.

112. Moo LR, Murphy KJ, Gailloud P, et al. Tailored cognitive testing with provocative amobarbital injection preceding AVM embolization. AJNR Am J Neuroradiol 2002;23:416–21.

113. Rauch RA, Vinuela F, Dion J, et al. Preembolization functional evaluation in brain arteriovenous malformations: the superselective Amytal test. AJNR Am J Neuroradiol 1992;13:303–8.

114. Gounis MJ, Lieber BB, Wakhloo AK, et al. Effect of glacial acetic acid and ethiodized oil concentration on embolization with N-butyl 2-cyanoacrylate: an in vivo investigation. AJNR Am J Neuroradiol 2002;23:938–44.

115. Jahan R, Murayama Y, Gobin YP, et al. Embolization of arteriovenous malformations with Onyx: clinicopathological experience in 23 patients. Neurosurgery 2001;48:984–95.

116. Chaloupka JC, Vinuela F, Vinters HV, et al. Technical feasibility and histopathologic studies of ethylene vinyl copolymer (EVAL) using a swine endovascular embolization model. AJNR Am J Neuroradiol 1994;15:1107–15.

117. Sampei K, Hashimoto N, Kazekawa K, et al. Histological changes in brain tissue and vasculature after intracarotid infusion of organic solvents in rats. Neuroradiology 1996;38:291–4.

118. Murayama Y, Vinuela F, Ulhoa A, et al. Nonadhesive liquid embolic agent for cerebral arteriovenous malformations: preliminary histopathological studies in swine rete mirabile. Neurosurgery 1998;43:1164–75.

119. Nogueira RG, Dabus G, Rabinov JD, et al. Preliminary experience with onyx embolization for the treatment of intracranial dural arteriovenous fistulas. AJNR Am J Neuroradiol 2008;29:91–7.

120. Yu SC, Chan MS, Lam JM, et al. Complete obliteration of intracranial arteriovenous malformation with endovascular cyanoacrylate embolization: initial success and rate of permanent cure. AJNR Am J Neuroradiol 2004;25:1139–43.

121. Yakes WF, Rossi P, Odink H. How I do it. Arteriovenous malformation management. Cardiovasc Intervent Radiol 1996;19:65–71.

122. Nakstad PH, Bakke SJ, Hald JK. Embolization of intracranial arteriovenous malformations and fistulas with polyvinyl alcohol particles and platinum fibre coils. Neuroradiology 1992;34:348–51.

123. Wakhloo AK, Juengling FD, Van Velthoven V, et al. Extended preoperative polyvinyl alcohol microembolization of intracranial meningiomas: assessment of two embolization techniques. AJNR Am J Neuroradiol 1993;14:571–82.

124. Mathis JA, Barr JD, Horton JA, et al. The efficacy of particulate embolization combined with stereotactic radiosurgery for treatment of large arteriovenous malformations of the brain. AJNR Am J Neuroradiol 1995;16:299–306.

125. Sorimachi T, Koike T, Takeuchi S, et al. Embolization of cerebral arteriovenous malformations achieved with polyvinyl alcohol particles: angiographic reappearance and complications. AJNR Am J Neuroradiol 1999;20:1323–8.

126. Deruty R, Pelissou-Guyotat I, Amat D, et al. Complications after multidisciplinary treatment of cerebral arteriovenous malformations. Acta Neurochir (Wien) 1996;138:119–31.

127. Pasqualin A, Scienza R, Cioffi F, et al. Treatment of cerebral arteriovenous malformations with a combination of preoperative embolization and surgery. Neurosurgery 1991;29:358–68.

128. Castel JP, Kantor G. [Postoperative morbidity and mortality after microsurgical exclusion of cerebral arteriovenous malformations. Current data and analysis of recent literature]. Neurochirurgie 2001; 47:369–83 [in French].

129. Jayaraman MV, Marcellus ML, Hamilton S, et al. Neurologic complications of arteriovenous malformation embolization using liquid embolic agents. AJNR Am J Neuroradiol 2008;29:242–6.

130. Aletich VA, Debrun GM. Intracranial arteriovenous malformations: the approach and technique of cyanoacrylate embolization. In: Connors JJ III, Wojak JC, editors. Interventional neuroradiology: strategies and practical techniques. Philadelphia: WB Saunders; 1999. p. 240–58.

131. Young WL, Pile-Spellman J. Anesthetic considerations for interventional neuroradiology. Anesthesiology 1994;80:427–56.

Neuroendovascular Management of Acute Ischemic Stroke

Stavropoula I. Tjoumakaris, MD*, Pascal M. Jabbour, MD,
Robert H. Rosenwasser, MD, FACS, FAHA

KEYWORDS

- Acute cerebrovascular accident
- Management • Endovascular • Stroke • Thrombolysis

Stroke is a major cause of serious, long-term disability and the third leading cause of death, after myocardial infarction and cancer. Approximately 800,000 strokes occur in the United States each year, leading to an estimated cost of $70 billion in 2009.[1] Management of acute ischemic stroke was previously geared toward prevention, supportive care, and rehabilitation. Over the past few decades, however, the medical management of stroke has progressed exponentially, beginning with the US Food and Drug Administration (FDA) approval of tissue plasminogen activator (r-TPA, alteplase) in 1996. Intravenous administration of r-TPA within a limited 3-hour window from symptom onset has shown a significant improvement in patient outcome at 3 months and at 1 year following an acute cerebrovascular event.[2]

The intra-arterial (IA) injection of therapeutic agents was first published nearly 60 years ago, when Sussman and Fitch[3] described the IA treatment of acute carotid occlusion with fibrinolysin injection in 1958. It was not until the late 1990s that the endovascular management of acute stroke experienced exponential progress and development. Recent advances in endovascular techniques have increased the therapeutic window of r-TPA administration and introduced new agents such as reteplase and abciximab. Furthermore, the use of IA devices for clot retrieval and vessel recanalization has revolutionized the neuroendovascular management of acute ischemic stroke.

PATIENT SELECTION

The goal of endovascular management of acute ischemic stroke is to enhance the survival of local ischemic brain tissue (penumbra) and limit the extent of infarcted brain parenchyma. An initial evaluation with a noncontrast computerized tomography (CT) head scan is necessary. Patients with large territorial infarcts on CT scan are at a higher risk for hemorrhagic conversion following treatment and are therefore poor candidates for endovascular therapy.[4] In addition, the presence of an intraparenchymal hematoma is a contraindication to endovascular recanalization. Last, the presence of a hyperdense middle cerebral artery (MCA) sign on the initial head CT does not have a significant prognostic value in patient outcome and vessel recanalization rates.[5–7]

Over the past decade, the clinical application of CT perfusion scans has facilitated the pretreatment evaluation of "salvageable" tissue. A scan consistent with a mismatch between cerebral blood volume (CBV, "core" cerebral lesion volume) and cerebral blood flow or mean transient time (CBF or MTT, "penumbra" lesion volume) is a favorable patient selection criterion.[8] In our institution, a favorable CT perfusion scan may overcome the 6-hour postsymptom-onset time restriction.

Although patient age and initial National Institutes of Health Stroke Scale score (NIHSS) do not show statistically significant correlation with

This article did not receive funding support.
Department of Neurological Surgery, Thomas Jefferson University, Jefferson Hospital for Neuroscience, 909 Walnut Street 3rd Floor, Philadelphia, PA 19107, USA
* Corresponding author.
E-mail address: stavropoula@gmail.com (S.I. Tjoumakaris).

Neurosurg Clin N Am 20 (2009) 419–429
doi:10.1016/j.nec.2009.07.005
1042-3680/09/$ – see front matter. Published by Elsevier Inc.

posttreatment intracranial hemorrhage (ICH), careful attention should be paid to both.[4] Furthermore, patient comorbidities are evaluated before treatment. Specifically, the presence of hyperglycemia, defined as blood sugar levels greater than 200 mg/dL within 24 hours from presentation, can significantly increase the likelihood of post-thrombolysis hemorrhagic conversion.[4]

Previous administration of intravenous tissue plasminogen activator is not a contraindication to IA intervention. However, the hemorrhagic complications in these patients are significantly higher, especially if urokinase was the arterial agent.[4] One must therefore clearly explain the risks and benefits of the procedure to the family and include them in the decision-making process. Overall, endovascular intervention is an invaluable tool in the management of acute ischemic stroke. However, the duration of ischemia and the presence of viable ischemic tissue in excess of irreversibly damaged tissue are both critical factors in the successful management of acute stroke.

ANGIOGRAPHIC EVALUATION

Initial angiographic evaluation of the patient's vasculature is of paramount importance for the establishment of the ischemic etiology and initiation of treatment. Femoral access is established in the symptomatic lower extremity, if no vascular contraindications exist. A thorough examination of the cerebrovascular anatomy begins with the aortic arch. The brachiocephalic vessels are visualized and any proximal stenosis, irregularities, or occlusion noted. Proximal vessel disease may require immediate treatment with balloon angioplasty and/or stenting to allow access to the intracranial pathology or may itself be the cause of the acute ischemic event.

Based on patient symptomatology and preprocedure imaging, selective catheterization of the carotid or vertebrobasilar circulation supplying the affected territory is performed. Attention is paid to the extracranial collateral circulation, the leptomeningeal anatomy, the circle of Willis, and overall global cerebral perfusion.

The modality of treatment (for example IA thrombolysis, balloon angioplasty, stenting, clot retrieval mechanisms) is tailored to each individual case. At times, advanced age or significant atherosclerotic disease may limit treatment options.

INTRA-ARTERIAL CHEMICAL THROMBOLYSIS

Over the past decade, several agents have been investigated for IA thrombolysis with variable dosages and administration routes. Overall, these drugs act by activating plasminogen to plasmin, which in turn degrades fibrin and its associated derivatives. Although studies targeting direct comparisons of the different agents have not yet been published, fibrin-specific agents, such as recombinant tissue plasminogen activator (r-tPA) and recombinant pro-urokinase (rpro-UK) have been widely studied and used most frequently.[9]

First-generation agents, such as streptokinase and urokinase, are nonfibrin selective and could therefore have greater systemic complications.[10] Streptokinase, a protein derivative from group C beta-hemolytic streptococci, has a half-life of 16 to 90 minutes. It has an increased association with intracranial and systemic hemorrhages, and was therefore removed from the chemical armamentarium for the management of acute ischemic stroke.[11] Urokinase, a serine protease, has a half-life of 14 minutes and dosage range of 0.02 to 2.00 million units.[12]

Second-generation agents have higher fibrin specificity and are most commonly studied in IA stroke management studies. Alteplase (r-tPA), also a serine protease, has a half-life of 3.5 minutes and a dosage range of 20 to 60 mg.[12] The precursor of urokinase (rpro-UK) has a half-life of 7 minutes and may be favorable to r-tPA because of decreased side effects. Kaur and colleagues[13] published potential neurotoxic properties of alteplase, such as activation of the N-methyl-D-aspartate (NMDA) receptor in the neuronal cell-death pathway, amplification of calcium conductance, and activation of extracellular matrix metalloproteinases. These effects may facilitate exacerbation of cerebral edema, disturbance of the blood brain barrier, and development of ICH.

Third-generation agents, such as reteplase and tenecteplase, have longer half-lives (15 to 18 minutes) and theoretically favorable vessel recanalization and local recurrence rates.[10] Newer-generation agents are genetically engineered, such as Desmoteplase and Microplasmin (Thrombogenics, Heverlee, Belgium).

Besides their fibrinolytic properties, the aforementioned agents have prothrombotic effects by the production of thrombin during thrombolysis, and subsequent activation of platelets and fibrinogen.[10] As a result, concomitant use of systemic anticoagulation during IA thrombolysis is recommended with caution to risk of ICH. The most widely used adjuvant systemic agent is heparin. Newer-generation agents under the category of glycoprotein (GP) IIIb/IIa antagonist, such as Reopro (abciximab) and Integrilin (eptifibatide) are currently under investigation.

ANTERIOR CIRCULATION
Middle Cerebral Artery

Three major clinical trials evaluated the efficacy of IA thrombolysis in the MCA circulation, specifically the PROACT I and II (Prolyse in Acute Cerebral Thromboembolism), and MELT trials (Middle Cerebral Artery Local Fibrinolytic Intervention Trial). Although IA thrombolysis shows a favorable outcome in the setting of acute ischemic injury, FDA approval has thus far been granted for its intravenous counterpart alone.[14]

In 1998, del Zoppo and colleagues[15] presented a phase II clinical trial investigating the safety and efficacy of IA delivery of rpro-UK in acute MCA stroke, PROACT I. Following the exclusion of intracranial hemorrhage with a noncontrast head CT, 40 patients were randomized for treatment of acute ischemic stroke within 6 hours of symptom onset. Cerebral angiography was performed, and M1 or M2 occlusions were treated with 6 mg of rpro-UK (n = 26) or placebo (n = 14). All patients received a concomitant heparin bolus followed by a 4-hour infusion. The final end points were recanalization efficacy at the end of the infusion period and neurologic deterioration from ICH within 24 hours of treatment. Rpro-UK treated patients had higher vessel recanalization rates compared with placebo (57.7% vs 14.3%). Furthermore, the incidence of ICH was higher in the rpro-UK group (15.4% vs 7.1%). Overall, PROACT I was the first organized trial proving the safety and efficacy of IA thrombolysis for the management of acute ischemic stroke.

PROACT II was a subsequent phase III clinical trial that studied the safety and efficacy of rpro-UK in a larger patient population (n = 180).[16] This randomized, controlled clinical trial treated patients with MCA occlusion within 6 hours of symptom onset with either 9 mg of IA rpro-UK and heparin infusion (n = 121) or heparin infusion alone (n = 59). The study's primary end point was the 90-day patient neurologic disability based on the modified Rankin score scale. Secondary outcomes included mortality, vessel recanalization, and neurologic deterioration from the development of ICH. Patients who received IA rpro-UK had significantly lower Rankin scores at the 90-day endpoint compared with heparin-only treated patients. Furthermore, the MCA recanalization and mortality rates favored the rpro-UK group as opposed to the control group (66% vs 18%). Albeit a higher incidence of ICH in the rpro-UK group (10% as opposed to 2% in the control group), the PROACT II multicenter trial demonstrated that the use of IA chemical thrombolysis in acute

ischemia of the anterior circulation leads to radiographic and clinical improvement.

Recently, the MELT Japanese study group investigated the IA administration of UK in the setting of MCA stroke within 6 hours of onset.[17] Although the study showed favorable 90-day functional outcome in the UK-treated patients with respect to controls, results did not reach statistical significance. Unfortunately, the investigation was aborted prematurely following the approval of intravenous r-TPA in Japan for the treatment of acute ischemic stroke.

The optimal window for IA thrombolysis in the anterior circulation has been investigated in multiple clinical trials. Overall, results show that IA treatment of acute MCA infarction outweighs potential hemorrhagic risks when implemented within a 6-hour window from symptom onset.[9] Theron and colleagues[18] investigated the efficacy of IA thrombolysis in patients with acute internal carotid artery (ICA) occlusion as it related to the timing of treatment and angiographic location. Based on their work, IA fibrinolysis of the MCA should be performed within 6 hours from ischemia onset, when the occlusion involves the horizontal segment of the MCA extending into the lenticulostriate arteries. Treatment complications, mainly hemorrhagic incidence, increase significantly beyond this optimal time frame. However, if the occlusion does not involve the horizontal MCA segment and the lenticulostriate arteries, then the treatment window can be extended to 12 hours following symptoms.[9] The paucity of collateral circulation in the lenticulostriate arteries, as well as their distal distribution, both contribute to their sensitivity to ischemia in the setting of acute stroke. When initiating endovascular intra-arterial thrombolysis, the operator should account for time required to perform the procedure. Considering that the average intervention time varies from 45 to 180 minutes, high-risk patients should be treated within 4 to 5 hours from ischemia onset.[19–21]

Internal Carotid Artery

Occlusions of the proximal ICA (extra-cranial) generally have a better prognosis than intracranial occlusions. The presence of external-internal carotid collateral flow and the anastomosis at the circle of Willis account for this observation. Patients with insufficient extracranial-intracranial anastomoses or an incomplete circle of Willis may be predisposed to developing significant neurologic symptoms. These patients are potential candidates for IA intervention. In these cases, mechanical thrombolysis, in addition to pharma-cologic thrombolysis, is of paramount importance for recanalization. In a 25-patient series, Jovin and colleagues[22] demonstrated successful revascular-ization in 92% of patients following thrombolysis and ICA stenting.

Intracranial ICA acute occlusions have a dismal natural history and overall prognosis. Negative prognostic factors include distal ICA distribution involving the M1 and A1 segments ("T" occlusion) and poor neurologic presentation. Arnold and colleagues[23] presented a series of 24 patients with distal ICA occlusions treated with IA urokinase. Favorable 3-month functional outcome was present in only 16% of patients, and the mortality rate was approximately 42%. Adjuvant mechanical assistance with devices for balloon angioplasty, clot retrieval, and vessel stenting enhance the probability of vessel recanalization (**Fig. 1**). Flint and colleagues[24] published a series of 80 patients with ICA occlusion who were treated with combina-tions of the Merci retriever (Concentric Medical, Mountain View, CA) with or without adjunctive en-dovascular therapy. Recanalization rates were higher in the combination group (63%) as opposed to the Merci group (53%). At a 3-month follow-up, 25% of patients had a good neurologic outcome, with their age being a positive predictive indicator. Overall, these results are encouraging, and IA inter-vention in select cases of acute ICA occlusion should be considered.

Central Retinal Artery

Occlusion of the central retinal artery (CRA) is an ophthalmologic emergency with a natural history that leads to loss of vision. Conventional medical therapy includes ocular massage, carbohydrate inhibitors, inhalation of carbogen mixture, para-centesis, topical beta-blockers, aspirin, and intra-venous heparin.[9] However, the limited efficacy of all these therapies made acute CRA occlusion a potential candidate for endovascular management.

Several studies have documented successful vessel recanalization with visual improvement compared with controls. In most studies, IA alte-plase is most commonly used within 4 to 6 hours from symptom onset. The agent is infused via superselective catheterization of the ophthalmic artery. Padolecchia and colleagues[25] showed that intervention within 4.5 hours of ischemic onset leads to visual improvement in all patients. Studies performed by Arnold and colleagues,[26] Aldrich and colleagues,[27] and Noble and colleagues[28] showed visual improvement in a significant number of patients treated with IA thrombolysis

that ranged from 22% to 93% compared with much lower conventionally treated controls. The IA agent was r-tPA or urokinase and the treatment time varied from 6 to 15 hours from symptom onset. Ischemic and hemorrhagic complications were either not present (Arnold and colleagues,[26] Aldrich and colleagues[27]) or occurred at signifi-cantly low rates (Noble and colleagues[28]).

POSTERIOR CIRCULATION

Acute basilar artery (BA) occlusion is a life-threat-ening event that poses a significant therapeutic challenge. The natural progression of untreated BA occlusion has mortality rates ranging from 86% to 100%.[9] The rare incidence of this disease, fewer than 10% of acute ischemic strokes, could account for the lack of significant randomized controlled studies in the topic. Several meta-anal-yses of case reports and case series reflect the severity of the disease. In a series of nearly 300 patients, Furlan and Higashida[29] reported an IA recanalization rate of 60%, and mortality rates of 31% in at least partially recanalized patients as opposed to 90% in non-recanalized patients. Lindsberg and Mattle compared BA occlusion treatment with intravenous (IV) or IA thrombolysis. They found that although recanalization rates were higher with IA treatment (65% vs 53%), depen-dency or death rates were equal between the two groups (76% to 78%). Overall, 22% of treated patients had good outcomes, as opposed to only 2% of untreated individuals. Therefore, emergent thrombolysis via either technique is of paramount importance to the survival of this patient population.

The timing of treatment initiation in relation to symptom onset is a controversial topic. Theoreti-cally, the same treatment restrictions apply as in the anterior circulation; however, in practice, the therapeutic window can be successfully extended beyond 6 hours. In our institution, we have achieved favorable clinical outcomes in patients treated up to 12 hours from symptom onset. Between 12 and 18 hours, incidence of hemor-rhagic conversion is more significant, and treat-ment is rarely extended beyond the 24-hour window. In the Basilar Artery International Cooper-ation Study (BASICS), 624 patients with radio-graphically confirmed occlusion of the BA were enrolled in nearly 50 centers over a 5-year period.[30] All patients (n = 41) treated with IA or IV thrombolytics beyond 9 hours from symptom onset had a poor reported outcome.

Recent advances in mechanical and pharmaco-logic approaches to endovascular therapies may increase BA recanalization rates and improve

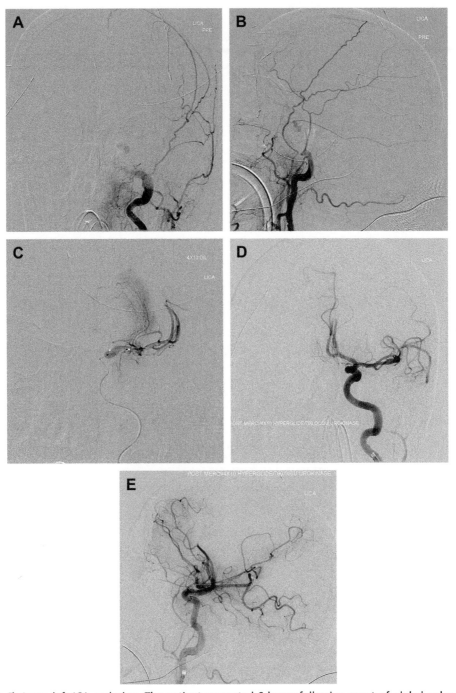

Fig. 1. (*A–E*) Acute left ICA occlusion. The patient presented 6 hours following onset of global aphasia and R hemiplegia. (*A, B*) Midarterial digital subtraction angiogram of left ICA artery showing complete occlusion of the distal ICA (T occlusion), frontal and lateral views. (*C*) Frontal view of balloon angioplasty and recanalization of the distal left ICA. (*D, E*) Frontal and lateral views of left ICA angiograms following mechanical and chemical recanalization with balloon angioplasty, Merci device, and administration of urokinase.

patient outcome (**Fig. 2**). In a meta-analysis of 164 patients with BA occlusion over a 10-year period, Levy and colleagues[31] reported several predictive factors in treatment consideration. Factors with a negative prognostic value were coma at initial presentation, failure of vessel recanalization, and proximal vessel occlusion. Distal BA occlusions are more commonly embolic in nature and therefore have a better response to thrombolytic agents.

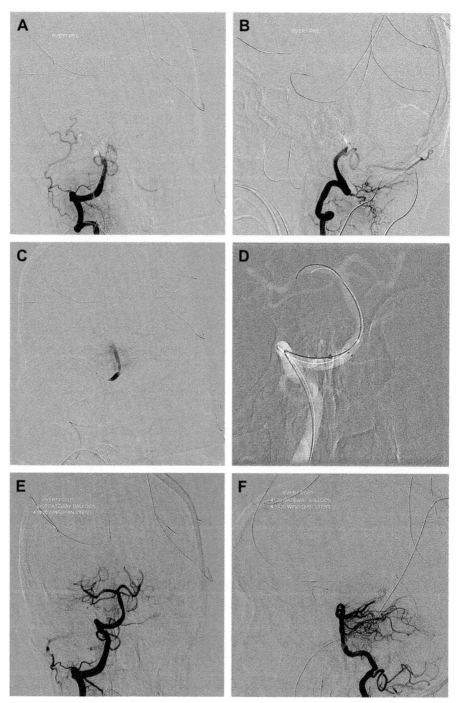

Fig. 2. (*A–F*) Acute right vertebro-basilar occlusion. (*A, B*) Midarterial digital subtraction angiogram of the right vertebral artery (dominant) showing complete occlusion with no distal filling of the basilar artery, frontal and lateral views. (*C*) Frontal view of balloon angioplasty of the right vertebro-basilar junction. (*D*) Road map during deployment of Wingspan stent at the vertebro-basilar level. (*E, F*) Frontal and lateral views of right vertebral artery midarterial angiograms depicting vessel recanalization following mechanical thrombolysis.

INTRA-ARTERIAL MECHANICAL THROMBOLYSIS

The use of mechanical endovascular devices for thrombolysis is emerging as a powerful adjuvant, or even an alternative to chemical thrombolysis. The mechanical disruption of the arterial clot has several advantages to IA management of acute stroke.[10] First, it increases the working surface area for thrombolytic agents thereby enhancing their efficacy. Even partial removal of clot via retrieval or thromboaspiration techniques lessens the concentration of IA agent required to dissolve the remainder pieces. As a result, the risk of ICH is further decreased and the treatment window could be extended beyond the 6-hour limit. Mechanical thrombolysis provides patients with contraindications to anticoagulation with a reasonable alternative to endovascular therapy.

The use of mechanical thrombolysis is associated with several associated risks. The endovascular trauma to the blood vessel could cause endothelial damage, permanent vascular injury, and ultimately vessel rupture, especially in old friable vessels. The technical skills needed for the endovascular navigation of such devices, especially through severely occluded segments, are substantial, and require rigorous training. Finally, the dislodged clot material could become an embolic source, exposing the already compromised distal circulation to additional ischemic risks.

Overall, the multiple advantages of mechanical endovascular devices have revolutionized current therapies of acute ischemic stroke, and are safe adjuvant and/or alternatives to chemical thrombolysis in experienced hands. The conceptual basis of such devices can be broadly categorized into the following categories: thrombectomy, thromboaspiration, thrombus disruption, augmented fibrinolysis, and thrombus entrapment.[10]

Endovascular Thrombectomy

Devices under this category apply a constant force to the clot material at its proximal or distal end and facilitate clot removal. Proximal end forces are applied through grasplike attachments, whereas distal end forces are applied via basketlike devices. The advantage of these devices is their decreased association with embolic material, as there is no attempt for mechanical clot disruption. Some of the most widely used examples are the Merci retriever (Concentric Medical), the Neuronet device (Guidant, Santa Clara, CA), the Phenox clot retriever (Phenox, Bochum, Germany), the Catch thrombectomy device (Balt Extrusion, Montmorency, France), and the Alligator retrieval device (Chestnut Medical Technologies, Menlo Park,

CA).[10] The Merci device became FDA approved in 2004 for endovascular clot retrieval in acute ischemic stroke.[32] It is a flexible nitinol wire with coil loops that incorporate into the clot and facilitate retrieval. In a recent study that investigated the efficacy of current thrombectomy mechanisms, the Merci, Phenox, and Catch devices presented equal results with clot mobilization and retrieval.[33]

Endovascular Thromboaspiration

The functioning mechanism in this category uses an aspiration technique, which is suited for fresh nonadhesive clots. These devices also have the advantage of less embolic material and decreased vasospasm. Some examples in this category are the Penumbra system (Penumbra, Alameda, CA) and the AngioJet system (Possis Medical, Minneapolis, MN).[10] The Penumbra system includes a reperfusion catheter that aspirates the clot and a ring-shaped retriever (**Fig. 3**). The favorable results of a prospective multicenter trial conducted in the United States and Europe led to the approval of the device by the FDA for the endovascular treatment of acute ischemic stroke in 2008.[34] The AngioJet system uses a high-pressure saline jet for clot agitation and an aspiration catheter for retrieval. Technical difficulties with endovascular navigation resulting in vessel injury led to the premature discontinuation of its trial in acute ischemic stroke patients.[35]

Thrombus Disruption

In this category, mechanical disruption of the clot is accomplished via a microguidewire or a snare. Some devices using this mechanism are the EPAR (Endovasix, Belmont, CA) and the LaTIS laser device (LaTIS, Minneapolis, MN).[10] The potential endothelial damage with resultant vessel injury and genesis of embolic material make these devices less favorable in the setting of acute ischemic stroke.

Augmented Fibrinolysis

These devices, such as the MicroLysUS infusion catheter (EKOS, Bothell, WA), use a sonographic micro-tip to facilitate thrombolysis through ultrasonic vibration.[10] As a result, clot removal is augmented without any additional fragment embolization to the distal circulation. Recent studies show a favorable outcome with the use of such devices for the endovascular management of acute ischemic stroke.[36,37]

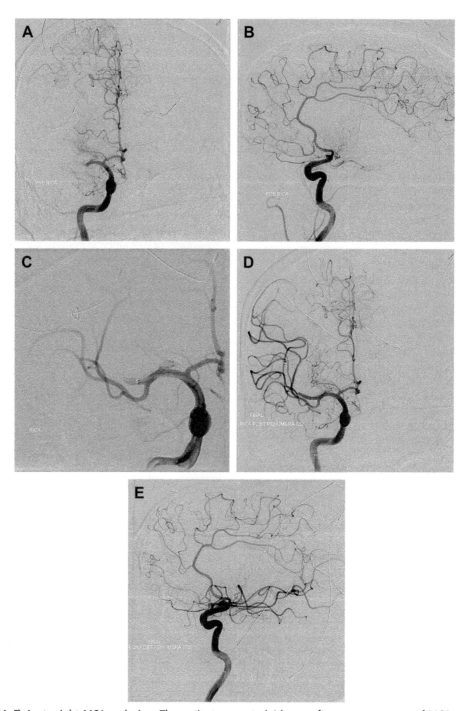

Fig. 3. (*A–E*) Acute right MCA occlusion. The patient presented 4 hours after an acute event of MCA occlusion. (*A, B*) Midarterial digital subtraction angiogram of right ICA shows complete MCA occlusion at the level of the bifurcation, frontal and lateral views. (*C*) Mechanical thrombolysis with Penumbra device showing recanalization of the superior M2 division in a frontal high-magnification view. (*D, E*) Frontal and lateral views of right ICA angiograms following MCA mechanical recanalization.

Thrombus Entrapment

The underlying mechanism of these devices uses a stent to recanalize the occluded vessel and therefore trap the clot between the stent and vessel wall. Besides their use at the site of occlusion, stents could recanalize proximal vessels (such as the extracranial ICA) to allow device navigation to the site of pathology. Stents can be deployed via a balloon mechanism or could be self-expandable. The latter are becoming increasingly popular because of their flexibility and ease of navigation. They include the Neuroform stent (Boston Scientific, Natick, MA), the Enterprise stent (Cordis, Miami Lakes, FL), the LEO stent (Balt Extrusion), the Solitaire/Solo stent (ev3, Irvine, CA), and the Wingspan stent (Boston Scientific). The first four stents are used in stent-assisted coiling of wide-neck aneurysms, whereas the Wingspan is the only stent approved for intracranial treatment of atherosclerotic disease.[10] Their use in acute ischemic events has been investigated in several trials. In two studies investigating the Neuroform and Wingspan stents, recanalization rates ranged from 67% to 89% and early follow-up (mean of 8 months) showed small (5%) or no restenosis rates.[38,39]

ALTERNATIVE REPERFUSION STRATEGIES

Cerebral reperfusion during acute ischemic stroke can be augmented via alternative strategies that use an anterograde or retrograde route. Anterograde reperfusion can be facilitated systemically with vasopressors leading to global reperfusion by increasing the mean arterial blood pressure. Retrograde reperfusion can be facilitated with a transarterial or transvenous approach. The transarterial approach involves the endovascular deployment of the NeuroFlo device (CoAxia, Maple Grove, MN). This dual balloon catheter allows for partial occlusion of the aorta above and below the level of the renal arteries, therefore diverting flow away from the systemic and toward the cerebral circulation.[40] Several clinical trials are currently under way investigating the safety and efficacy of NeuroFlo and similar devices.

Transvenous retrograde reperfusion is an experimental technique with potential benefit in acute ischemic stroke. Animal studies suggest that diversion of blood from the femoral artery into the transverse venous sinuses via transvenous catheters could lower infarction size and improve neurologic outcome in the setting of acute cerebrovascular ischemia.[41] Further investigational human trials are required before introducing such a novel concept to current stroke therapies.

FUTURE DIRECTIONS

Advances in knowledge about pharmacology, endovascular biomechanics, and endothelial properties are stimulating research on new diagnostic and therapeutic tools in the management of acute ischemic stroke. Currently there are several clinical trials targeting neuroendovascular therapy.[14] The Interventional Management of Stroke Study III (IMS III) is a phase III multicenter clinical trial that continues the investigation of combined IA and IV therapies in the management of acute stroke. The SYNTHESIS Expansion trial is a phase III clinical study that compares the safety and efficacy of IV thrombolysis to IA chemical and mechanical thrombolysis.

Multiple studies are investigating the safety and efficacy of new-generation endovascular devices, such as the Safety and Efficacy of NeuroFlo Technology in Ischemic Stroke (SENTIS). The neurologic outcomes of optimal medical management versus IA thrombolysis are examined in clinical trials such as RETRIEVE (Randomized Trial of Endovascular treatment of Acute Ischemic Stroke Versus Medical Management) and PISTE (Pragmatic Ischemic Stroke Thrombectomy Evaluation). Extending the timing of endovascular intervention is being evaluated in conjunction with new radiographic techniques. Examples include the DWI and CTP Assessment in the Triage of Wake-Up and Late Presenting Strokes Undergoing Neurointervention Trial, and the MR Imaging and Recanalization of Stroke Clots During Embolectomy Trial.[14]

These and several other upcoming trials will hopefully provide sufficient clinical data for the FDA approval of IA agents, the introduction of new endovascular devices, and other adjunctive therapies for the management of the acute stroke patient.

SUMMARY

The preponderance of data shows that endovascular intervention has become a mainstay treatment in the setting of acute ischemic stroke, and will continue to evolve. Innovative techniques in both chemical and mechanical intra-arterial thrombolysis increase the safety and efficacy of endovascular management and expand its indications in acute cerebral infarction. Additional larger clinical trials are warranted for the improvement of the endovascular care of stroke patients resulting in faster and safer reperfusion mechanisms.

REFERENCES

1. AHA. Heart and Stroke Update. 2009.

2. Fagan SC, Morgenstern LB, Petitta A, et al. Cost-effectiveness of tissue plasminogen activator for acute ischemic stroke. NINDS rt-PA Stroke Study Group. Neurology 1998;50:883–90.

3. Sussman BJ, Fitch TS. Thrombolysis with fibrinolysin in cerebral arterial occlusion. JAMA 1958;167: 1705–9.

4. Vora NA, Gupta R, Thomas AJ, et al. Factors predicting hemorrhagic complications after multimodal reperfusion therapy for acute ischemic stroke. AJNR Am J Neuroradiol 2007;28:1391–4.

5. Gönner F, Remonda L, Mattle H, et al. Local intra-arterial thrombolysis in acute ischemic stroke. Stroke 1998;29:1894–900.

6. von Kummer R, Meyding-Lamadé U, Forsting M, et al. Sensitivity and prognostic value of early CT in occlusion of the middle cerebral artery trunk. AJNR Am J Neuroradiol 1994;15:9–15 [discussion: 16–8].

7. Wolpert SM, Bruckmann H, Greenlee R, et al. Neuroradiologic evaluation of patients with acute stroke treated with recombinant tissue plasminogen activator. The rt-PA Acute Stroke Study Group. AJNR Am J Neuroradiol 1993;14:3–13.

8. Konstas AA, Goldmakher GV, Lee TY, et al. Theoretic basis and technical implementations of CT perfusion in acute ischemic stroke, part 1: theoretic basis. AJNR Am J Neuroradiol 2009;30:662–8.

9. Berenstein Alejandro, Lasjaunias Pierre, G. ter Brugge Karel. Surgical neuroangiography. Clinical and endovascular treatment. 2nd edition. Springer; 2004.

10. Nogueira RG, Schwamm LH, Hirsch JA. Endovascular approaches to acute stroke, part 1: drugs, devices, and data. AJNR Am J Neuroradiol 2009; 30:649–61.

11. Cornu C, Boutitie F, Candelise L, et al. Streptokinase in acute ischemic stroke: an individual patient data meta-analysis: the thrombolysis in acute stroke pooling project. Stroke 2000;31:1555–60.

12. Lisboa RC, Jovanovic BD, Alberts MJ. Analysis of the safety and efficacy of intra-arterial thrombolytic therapy in ischemic stroke. Stroke 2002;33:2866–71.

13. Kaur J, Zhao Z, Klein GM, et al. The neurotoxicity of tissue plasminogen activator? J Cereb Blood Flow Metab 2004;24:945–63.

14. Nogueira RG, Yoo AJ, Buonanno FS, et al. Endovascular approaches to acute stroke, part 2: a comprehensive review of studies and trials. AJNR Am J Neuroradiol 2009;30:859–75.

15. del Zoppo GJ, Higashida RT, Furlan AJ, et al. A phase II randomized trial of recombinant pro-urokinase by direct arterial delivery in acute middle cerebral artery stroke. PROACT Investigators. Prolyse in Acute Cerebral Thromboembolism. Stroke 1998;29: 4–11.

16. Furlan A, Higashida R, Wechsler L, et al. Intra-arterial prourokinase for acute ischemic stroke. The PROACT II study: a randomized controlled trial. Prolyse in acute cerebral thromboembolism. JAMA 1999;282:2003–11.

17. Ogawa A, Mori E, Minematsu K, et al. Randomized trial of intraarterial infusion of urokinase within 6 hours of middle cerebral artery stroke: the middle cerebral artery embolism local fibrinolytic intervention trial (MELT) Japan. Stroke 2007;38:2633–9.

18. Theron J, Courtheoux P, Casasco A, et al. Local intraarterial fibrinolysis in the carotid territory. AJNR Am J Neuroradiol 1989;10:753–65.

19. Brott T. Thrombolytic therapy. Neurol Clin 1992;10: 219–32.

20. Levine SR, Brott TG. Thrombolytic therapy in cerebrovascular disorders. Prog Cardiovasc Dis 1992; 34:235–62.

21. Barnwell SL, Clark WM, Nguyen TT, et al. Safety and efficacy of delayed intraarterial urokinase therapy with mechanical clot disruption for thromboembolic stroke. AJNR Am J Neuroradiol 1994;15:1817–22.

22. Jovin TG, Gupta R, Uchino K, et al. Emergent stenting of extracranial internal carotid artery occlusion in acute stroke has a high revascularization rate. Stroke 2005;36:2426–30.

23. Arnold M, Nedeltchev K, Mattle HP, et al. Intra-arterial thrombolysis in 24 consecutive patients with internal carotid artery T occlusions. J Neurol Neurosurg Psychiatr 2003;74:739–42.

24. Flint AC, Duckwiler GR, Budzik RF, et al. Mechanical thrombectomy of intracranial internal carotid occlusion: pooled results of the MERCI and Multi MERCI Part I trials. Stroke 2007;38:1274–80.

25. Padolecchia R, Puglioli M, Ragone MC, et al. Superselective intraarterial fibrinolysis in central retinal artery occlusion. AJNR Am J Neuroradiol 1999;20: 565–7.

26. Arnold M, Koerner U, Remonda L, et al. Comparison of intra-arterial thrombolysis with conventional treatment in patients with acute central retinal artery occlusion. J Neurol Neurosurg Psychiatr 2005;76: 196–9.

27. Aldrich EM, Lee AW, Chen CS, et al. Local intraarterial fibrinolysis administered in aliquots for the treatment of central retinal artery occlusion: the Johns Hopkins Hospital experience. Stroke 2008;39: 1746–50.

28. Noble J, Weizblit N, Baerlocher MO, et al. Intra-arterial thrombolysis for central retinal artery occlusion: a systematic review. Br J Ophthalmol 2008;92: 588–93.

29. Furlan A, Higashida R. Intra-arterial thrombolysis in acute ischemic stroke. Stroke: pathophysiology, diagnosis, and management. 4th edition. Philadelphia: Churchill Livingstone; 2004. p. 943–51.

30. Schonewille WJ, Wijman CA, Michel P, et al. The basilar artery international cooperation study (BASICS). Int J Stroke 2007;2:220–3.

31. Levy EI, Firlik AD, Wisniewski S, et al. Factors affecting survival rates for acute vertebrobasilar artery occlusions treated with intra-arterial thrombolytic therapy: a meta-analytical approach. Neurosurgery 1999;45:539–45 [discussion: 545–8].

32. Smith WS, Sung G, Starkman S, et al. Safety and efficacy of mechanical embolectomy in acute ischemic stroke: results of the MERCI trial. Stroke 2005;36: 1432–8.

33. Liebig T, Reinartz J, Hannes R, et al. Comparative in vitro study of five mechanical embolectomy systems: effectiveness of clot removal and risk of distal embolization. Neuroradiology 2008;50:43–52.

34. Bose A, Henkes H, Alfke K, et al. The Penumbra System: a mechanical device for the treatment of acute stroke due to thromboembolism. AJNR Am J Neuroradiol 2008;29:1409–13.

35. Nesbit GM, Luh G, Tien R, et al. New and future endovascular treatment strategies for acute ischemic stroke. J Vasc Interv Radiol 2004;15:S103–10.

36. Mahon BR, Nesbit GM, Barnwell SL, et al. North American clinical experience with the EKOS Micro-LysUS infusion catheter for the treatment of embolic stroke. AJNR Am J Neuroradiol 2003;24:534–8.

37. Investigators T II. The Interventional Management of Stroke (IMS) II Study. Stroke 2007;38:2127–35.

38. Levy EI, Mehta R, Gupta R, et al. Self-expanding stents for recanalization of acute cerebrovascular occlusions. AJNR Am J Neuroradiol 2007;28: 816–22.

39. Zaidat OO, Wolfe T, Hussain SI, et al. Interventional acute ischemic stroke therapy with intracranial self-expanding stent. Stroke 2008;39:2392–5.

40. Lylyk P, Vila JF, Miranda C, et al. Partial aortic obstruction improves cerebral perfusion and clinical symptoms in patients with symptomatic vasospasm. Neurol Res 2005;27(Suppl 1):S129–35.

41. Frazee JG, Luo X, Luan G, et al. Retrograde transvenous neuroperfusion: a back door treatment for stroke. Stroke 1998;29:1912–6.

Neuroendovascular Management of Dural Arteriovenous Malformations

Kathleen A. McConnell, MD[a], Stavropoula I. Tjoumakaris, MD[b],*,
Jason Allen, MD[a], Maksim Shapiro, MD[a],
Tibor Bescke, MD[c], Pascal M. Jabbour, MD[b],
Robert H. Rosenwasser, MD, FACS, FAHA[b,e,f], Peter K. Nelson, MD[a,d]

KEYWORDS

- Dural arteriovenous fistula • Endovascular
- Therapy • Arteriovenous shunt
- Dural arteriovenous malformation

Approximately 10% to 15% of all clinically apparent intracranial arteriovenous malformations (AVMs) are of the dural type and are frequently referred to as dural arteriovenous fistulas (dAVFs).[1] These lesions are characterized by discrete arteriovenous (AV) fistulas involving the intracranial venous sinuses or dural veins. Although the causes of most dural arteriovenous fistulas remain unknown, there is evidence that fistula formation is preceded in some instances by trauma resulting in skull fracture, sinus thromboses, or venous outlet stenoses, increasing antegrade downstream outflow impedance of the involved dural venous sinus.[2] In cases related to pre-existing sinus thrombosis, it has been postulated that during recanalization, a pathologic fistula develops, possibly from degenerative changes involving a normal physiologically regulated arteriovenous shunt or from the triggering of a latent congenital dural AV shunt that ultimately progresses to a clinically and angiographically apparent syndrome. With the exception of those shunts localizing to the posterior fossa, dAVFs are more prevalent in women and usually diagnosed in patients between the ages of 30 and 80 years.[3]

dAVFs are typically classified by location of the involved sinus or shunt and by the pattern of venous drainage.[2] The latter scheme allows the subdivision of dAVFs into five types found to correlate with clinical symptomatology. Type I dAVFs are characterized by a degree of arteriovenous shunting not exceeding the involved venous sinus segment's antegrade outflow capacity, resulting in exclusive ipsilateral extracranial drainage of the shunt. Type II dAVFs exhibit a degree of AV shunting exceeding the capacity of antegrade outflow from the involved sinus, resulting in retrograde venous drainage into the adjacent sinus segments (type IIa), cortical veins (type IIb), or both (type IIa + b). Types III and IV dAVFs drain directly into cortical veins, with (type IV) or without (type III)

[a] Department of Radiology, New York University Langone Medical Center, New York, NY, USA
[b] Department of Neurological Surgery, Thomas Jefferson University, Jefferson Hospital for Neuroscience, 909 Walnut Street, 3rd Floor, Philadelphia, PA 19107, USA
[c] Department of Neurology, New York University Langone Medical Center, New York, NY, USA
[d] Department of Neurosurgery, New York University Langone Medical Center, New York, NY, USA
[e] Department of Radiology, Thomas Jefferson University, Jefferson Hospital for Neuroscience, Philadelphia, PA, USA
[f] Division of Cerebrovascular Surgery and Interventional Neuroradiology, Thomas Jefferson University, Jefferson Hospital for Neuroscience, Philadelphia, PA, USA
* Corresponding author.
E-mail address: stavropoula@gmail.com (S.I. Tjoumakaris).

Neurosurg Clin N Am 20 (2009) 431–439
doi:10.1016/j.nec.2009.07.014
1042-3680/09/$ – see front matter. Published by Elsevier Inc.

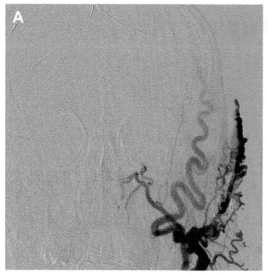
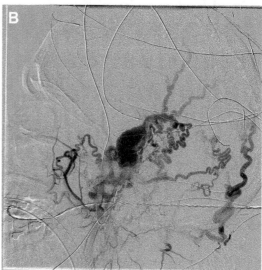

Fig. 1. Frontal (*A*) and lateral (*B*) unsubtracted views of left external carotid artery, showing a dAVF, with arterial feeders from left superficial temporal and occipital arteries. Note deep cortical venous drainage and a large venous aneurysm. Superficial temporal feeders have been partially embolized with Onyx.

venous ectasia (**Fig. 1**). Type V dAVFs are typically localized to the tentorium or dural coverings of the posterior fossa and are further characterized by drainage inferiorly into the intrathecal spinal veins. Types II and higher dAVFs are associated with a more aggressive natural history and, when technically feasible, are generally treated because of their increased risk of symptomatic presentation.

Recently, Geibprasert and colleagues[4] have proposed an ambitious classification, conceptually unifying pathophysiologic consequences of cranial and spinal dAVF on an embryologic basis. This scheme is based on the venous afferent patterns of three epidural spaces: (1) the ventral drainage group derived from the notochord and corresponding sclerotome extending from the base of the sphenoid to the sacrum; (2) the dorsal epidural space derived primarily from the dorsally located intracranial dural sinuses, because this space is not well developed in the spine; and (3) the lateral epidural shunts located where lateral pial emissary bridging veins pierce the dura. By examining 300 patients with dAVFs and categorizing their lesions by their respective afferent venous patterns, Geibprasert and colleagues were able to establish some clinical generalizations about each group. Ventral epidural shunts demonstrated a 2.3:1 female predominance and were less likely associated with cortical venous reflux unless there was extensive thrombosis of the epidural drainage or an especially high-flow shunt. Similarly, dorsal epidural shunts were less like to reflux into the cortical veins unless thrombosis was present. These lesions did not demonstrate sex predominance but did tend to occur in a lower age group (pediatric) and occur more frequently as multiple lesions. The lateral epidural shunts tended to present in older age groups and were more common in men. These lateral lesions were always clinically aggressive and demonstrated significant cortical venous reflux.

CLINICAL FEATURES OF DURAL ARTERIOVENOUS FISTULAS AND ANATOMIC CONSIDERATIONS FOR EMBOLIZATION

The clinical features associated with dAVFs generally depend on the location of the lesion, the extent of the AV shunting, and associated abnormalities of venous drainage.[1,5] Symptoms may be indistinguishable from those associated with pial brain AVMs and may include headache, diplopia, blurred vision, or neurologic dysfunction. Focal neurologic deficits and seizures may develop in relation to disturbances in regional cortical venous drainage resulting from the redirection of venous flow from the shunt into pial veins, potentially congesting venous territory remote from the site of the dural AVM. In patients with severe compromise of the deep venous drainage of the brain or with diffuse intracranial hypertension resulting from the obstruction of both sigmoid sinuses, clinical presentation may include dementia.[2] Closure of the arteriovenous shunts may successfully reverse this state only when there are adequate residual venous channels available for the normal venous drainage of the brain. Rarely, cranial neuropathy or unilateral visual phenomena may arise secondary to arterial steal without evidence of associated venous hypertension.[6] Focal symptomatology may worsen or change as a result of the redirection of venous outflow from a dAVF. For example, progressive thrombosis and occlusion of the inferior and superior petrosal sinuses may be associated with worsening of signs in patients with dAVFs of the cavernous sinus (CSdAVFs) draining anteriorly through the ipsilateral ophthalmic veins. If contralateral drainage is available, the venous sinus hypertension may be transmitted to the contralateral cavernous sinus, leading to development of bilateral orbital symptomatology.

The signs and symptoms of increased intracranial pressure occasionally complicate cases of dAVFs. In certain cases this can be attributed to diminished cerebrospinal fluid absorption through the arachnoid villi resulting from the transmission of increased venous pressure throughout the superior sagittal sinus. Alternatively, obstruction of the cerebral aqueduct secondary to compression of the mesencephalon by an ectatic draining vein may occur, leading to obstructive hydrocephalus.[7]

Moreover, aneurysmal venous ectasia may cause symptomatic mechanical compression of adjacent neurologic structures, most commonly in dAVFs draining into pial veins of the posterior fossa. This is particularly true for type IV dAVFs, which not infrequently present with clinical symptoms related to mass effect caused by pronounced venous ectasia.[2]

Approximately 20% to 33% of patients with symptomatic dAVFs present with an intracranial hemorrhage. This is encountered most frequently in lesions involving the floor of the anterior cranial fossa or the tentorium cerebelli; however, it may occur in any case associated with cortical venous drainage, particularly in the presence of significant cerebral venous ectasia.[2]

For those dAVFs that present in ways other than hemorrhage, the clinical presentation depends entirely on the grade, location, and venous afferent pattern of the fistula. This allows dAVFs to be categorized clinicoanatomically as those involving the cavernous sinus, transverse and sigmoid sinuses, superior sagittal sinus, petrosal sinus, torcular, tentorial incisura, and anterior cranial base.

Approximately one third to one half of symptomatic intracranial dAVFs involve the transverse and sigmoid sinuses (**Fig. 2**).[8] Patients with this condition often present with a subjective bruit as the first clinical manifestation. The tinnitus is synchronized to arterial pulsations and results from turbulence associated with the shunting of blood into the sigmoid or transverse sinuses. Auscultation over the retroauricular area usually reveals the pulsatile bruit. As with the other dAVFs, additional neurologic symptoms and findings generally depend on the pattern of venous drainage encountered in individual patients. Symptoms may include chronic signs of increased intracranial pressure potentially leading to papilledema and optic atrophy in addition to disturbances related to balance and hearing. In progressive cases, associated with obstruction of the ipsilateral jugular outflow, redirected venous drainage into pial veins of the posterior fossa may result in brain stem or cerebellar dysfunction and posterior fossa hemorrhage. Rerouting of drainage into the supratentorial cortical venous compartment may be associated with the development of focal neurologic deficit or seizures and increased risk of intracranial hemorrhage.

dAVFs involving the superior sagittal sinus, tentorial incisura, petrosal sinuses, and anterior cranial base occur less frequently than dAVFs involving the transverse, sigmoid, or cavernous sinuses.[2,9] In these lesions, symptoms typically depend on the route of abnormal venous drainage and associated pattern of venous hypertension and may include dysphasia, hemiparesis, hemisensory deficits, and abnormal visual phenomena. Following specific features deserve particular attention. (1) Dural fistulas involving the floor of the anterior cranial fossa are usually associated with drainage into ectatic parasagittal cortical veins and often present with intracranial hemorrhage.[9] Moreover, patients may exhibit unilateral visual loss secondary to arterial steal from the ophthalmic circulation into ethmoidal and recurrent meningeal supplies to the shunt. (2) dAVFs of the petrosal sinuses or tentorial incisura may occasionally drain inferiorly into perimedullary veins of the spinal cord (type V), resulting in progressive myelopathy similar to that encountered in spinal dural AVMs.[8] Assuming the venous sinus drainage of the brain is otherwise unimpaired, these symptoms usually respond well to endovascular or surgical closure of the shunt.

dAVFs most frequently involve the transverse sinuses. Arterial supply to fistulae of this region predictably derive from identifiable supratentorial and infratentorial sources. The supratentorial group is usually organized around (1) contributors to the basal tentorial arcade, typically including the petrosal and petrosquamosal divisions of the middle meningeal *artery* (MMA) and the lateral division of the meningohypophyseal trunk off the ICA, and, occasionally, (2) tranosseous branches of the posterior auricular artery. The infratentorial group commonly involves the jugular division of the ascending pharyngeal artery (APA), transmastoid

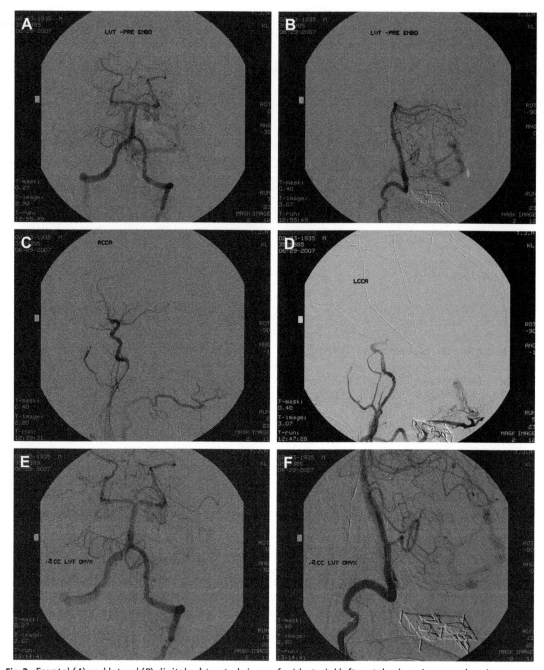

Fig. 2. Frontal (*A*) and lateral (*B*) digital subtracted views of midarterial left vertebral angiogram, showing a posterior fossa dAVF, with arterial feeders from left vertebral artery and deep cortical venous drainage. Lateral projections of right (*C*) and left (*D*) common carotid artery subtracted angiograms with bilateral occipital artery feeders to the dAVF. Frontal (*E*) and lateral (*F*) projections of left vertebral artery after Onyx dAVF embolization.

and more distal transosseous branches of the occipital artery, and the posterior meningeal arteries and artery of the falx cerebelli, either of which can variably arise from the occipital artery, vertebral artery, or APA or, rarely, directly from the posterior inferior cerebellar *artery*. With higher-flow lesions, indirect contribution from

contralateral sources may be seen but this usually involves anastomosis with one of the conduits (discussed previously) as a final common pathway.

In terms of embolization hazards, the petrosal branch of the MMA notably gives rise to a branch that anastomoses with the stylomastoid branch of the occipital or posterior auricular arteries, forming an arterial arcade within the facial canal, which, if aggressively embolized (inadvertently), may result in damage to the facial nerve. In that the petrosal branch of the MMA usually participates in the supply of transverse sinus dAVF through the basal tentorial arcade, its contribution to the lesion commonly can be indirectly devascularized by accessing the basal tentorial arcade posterolaterally through the petrosquamosal division of the MMA, avoiding the need for direct catheterization and embolization of the petrosal branch altogether. The basal tentorial arcade is an arterial network extending along the insertion of the tentorium into the petrous ridge from the petroclinoid ligament laterally to the transverse sinus. The jugular division of the APA enters the cranial vault via the jugular foramen supplying cranial nerves (CNs) 9, 10, and 11 before dividing into medial and lateral divisions. The medial division courses along the inferior petrosal sinus where it supplies CN 6 and anastamoses with the medial division of the lateral clival branch of MHT. The lateral division runs superiorly along the sigmoid sinus and vascularizes the dura along the transverse sigmoidal confluence. In very high–flow fistulae of the distal transverse sinus or lesions of the sigmoid sinus and foramen magnum, recruitment of supply through the hypoglossal division of the APA may be seen (particularly where this artery gives rise to the ipsilateral posterior meningeal artery). Transarterial embolizations through this division of the APA (particularly with liquid embolic agents) may result in injury to CN 12, leading to ipsilateral paresis of the tongue.

CSdAVFs are generally associated with orbital signs and symptoms that fluctuate depending on alterations in orbital venous outflow, which develop secondary to thrombosis and changes in head position. Patients typically present with the gradual onset of focal or diffuse chronic eye redness distinguishable from uveitis. Close inspection reveals dilated tortuous conjunctival and epibulbar vessels that exhibit an acute angulation near the ocular limbus.[10,11] These lesions are often associated with an elevation of episcleral venous pressure leading to a persistent rise in intraocular pressure in the affected eye, potentially resulting in the development of glaucoma. If both cavernous sinuses become involved in the venous drainage secondary to a change in the ipsilateral venous outflow of the affected cavernous sinus, the ocular findings may become bilateral. Patients may complain of pulsatile tinnitus, and in 25% of cases a bruit can be auscultated over the orbit.[2] Cranial neuropathies, most commonly involving the sixth nerve, frequently lead to ocular motor

dysfunction, which may be exacerbated by orbital venous congestion and proptosis. More important to the planning of embolization are the hypoxic ischemic retinal changes that develop in approximately 15% of patients.[1] Rarely, if thrombosis in the cavernous sinus is extensive, abnormal drainage into cerebral veins may occur, increasing the likelihood of an intracranial hemorrhage or venous infarction.[2] Unfortunately, frequently cited classification schemes of intracranial dAVFs are deficient in their handling of CSdAVFs due to the lack of explicit consideration given to ophthalmic venous drainage and the clinical consequences of orbital venous congestion. Despite the lack of a coherent classification scheme for CSdAVFs, the implications of venous outflow from these lesions are similar to dAVFs at other locations and the analysis of venous drainage is important in understanding the pathophysiology of the disease at this site. An excellent study of the clinical manifestations in 85 patients with CSdAVF relative to their angiographic characteristics was reported by Stiebel-Kalish and colleagues.[12,13] In this study, the clinical symptoms found in patients with CSdAVFs were related to the abnormal venous drainage and could be predicted by analysis of the aberrant venous drainage patterns. Central nervous system symptoms or dysfunction was found in seven (8%) of these patients, attesting to the potential danger of cortical venous drainage even among patients with CSdAVF.

The vascular supply to the dura of the cavernous sinus is complex because of extensive regional anastomoses between dural branches of the internal carotid and branches of the internal maxillary artery (middle meningeal and accessory meningeal arteries and the artery of the foramen rotundum). Moreover, the ophthalmic artery may participate indirectly via a tentorial branch of the recurrent meningeal artery. From the perspective of angiographic work-up and embolization, these lesions may be divided conceptually into two groups: (1) an anterolateral group, arising from the orbital apex and lateral cavernous sinus, and (2) a posterior group, including the posterior cavernous sinus, petroclinoid ligament, and dorsum sella.

The meningeal supply to anterior division lesions may be considered as reflecting the hemodynamic balance between branches arising from the horizontal segment of the cavernous internal carotid artery, most notably the inferolateral trunk and meningeal branches of the internal maxillary artery. This latter group includes cavernous and recurrent tentorial branches of the MMA, cavernous meningeal branches of the accessory meningeal artery, and the artery of the foramen rotundum. As expected, embolization of these meningeal arteries should be preceded by superselective angiographic analysis to prevent inadvertent embolization into the internal carotid artery or possible damage to the orbit or regional cranial nerves.

The supply to posterior division lesions is derived primarily from medial and lateral clival (meningohypophyseal) branches of the internal carotid artery and their potential anastomotic connections with branches of the APA and MMAs. These most notably include the ascending clival and inferior petrosal arcades, derived from the hypoglossal and jugular divisions of the APA, respectively; the posterior cavernous branches of the MMA; and the basal tentorial arcade supplied by the petrosal and the petrosquamosal branches of the MMA.

Three critical points should be considered before embolization of fistulae involving this territory. (1) The vascular supply to the intrapetrous facial nerve should be determined. Because supply may arise primarily from the petrous branch of the MMA, petroclinoid lesions supplied by the basal tentorial arcade should be embolized preferentially from the petrosquamosal branch of the MMA, thereby avoiding the proximal petrosal artery. (2) Potential contributions from the contralateral internal carotid pharyngeal artery and APA via transclival anastomoses should be evaluated, particularly in lesions involving the dorsum sellae. (3) Because embolization of upper clival and petroclinoid lesions may involve the hypoglossal or jugular division of the APA, attention must be directed to the possibility of iatrogenic lower cranial neuropathy when using N-butyl cyanoacrylate (NBCA), ethylene vinyl alcohol copolymer dissolved in dimethyl sulfoxide (Onyx), or ethanol. Midline lesions requiring aggressive embolization of pedicles from APAs should be performed as a staged procedure on different days, specifically to avoid development of bilateral hypoglossal nerve deficits.

NEUROIMAGING OF INTRACRANIAL DURAL ARTERIOVENOUS FISTULAS

Recent advances in CT and MRI have significantly contributed to the initial diagnostic evaluation of patients with suspected dAVFs. Although routine conventional head CT or brain MRI is not infrequently diagnostically equivocal, dilated or thrombosed venous structures suggesting the presence of a lesion may be identified, particularly in patients with dAVFs associated with cortical venous drainage. In patients presenting with intracranial hemorrhage, obvious findings are evident in CT and MRI studies. Focal or generalized atrophy of the brain, possibly accompanied by

hydrocephalus, are nonspecific secondary findings that may be appreciated. The chronic enlargement of meningeal branches of the external carotid or carotid-cavernous artery may be demonstrated by imaging studies. Despite the presence of secondary signs that suggest the presence of a dAVF, conventional MRI alone is generally unsuccessful in defining the exact site of fistualization.

The advent of CT angiography and magnetic resonance angiography (MRA) has provided more power to the noninvasive screening of patients with suspected dAVFs. In addition to providing anatomic details, these modalities may be coupled with perfusion studies to evaluate the effect of a dAVF on regional blood flow.

MRA may be performed using a three-dimensional time-of-flight (3D-TOF) technique or MR digital subtraction angiography (MR-DSA).[14–17] The presence of multiple high-intensity curvilinear or nodular structures adjacent to a sinus, in conjunction with high-intensity foci within the sinus, is considered suspicious for a dAVF; however, the technique still suffers from a high false-positive rate, with as many as 14% of otherwise healthy patients incorrectly identified as possibly harboring a dAVF by 3D-TOF MRA. Although the current spatial resolution of MR-DSA is less than 3D-TOF MRA, the benefit of MR-DSA is related to the temporal resolution of the technique and the ability to depict flow within cortical veins, which are particularly important in those patients with retrograde flow from a dAVF.

Despite advances in CT angiography and MRA, conventional DSA remains paramount in the diagnosis and pretreatment analysis of intracranial dAVFs. The angiographic evaluation usually includes selective studies of the internal and external carotid arteries bilaterally and of both vertebral arteries when evaluating lesions of the posterior fossa or tentorium. The pretherapeutic examination must be tailored to the clinically suspected location of the fistula and must disclose the entire arterial supply and any anastomoses between the supplying vessels and arterial distributions to the orbit, brain, or cranial nerves. This usually requires superselective arterial catheterization and angiography before the use of embolic materials. The venous anatomy must be studied with respect to the pattern of drainage from the fistula, and the adequacy of normal venous drainage of the brain must be assessed.

THERAPEUTIC APPROACHES TO DURAL ARTERIOVENOUS FISTULAS

An understanding of the natural history of the disease, the treatment options, and the risks and benefits of endovascular therapies is important in the development of a treatment plan. Although spontaneous resolution of clinical signs related to dAVFs has been reported, most notably in patients with cavernous sinus lesions, most symptomatic dAVFs require some form of treatment. This is most urgent in those fistulas accompanied by cortical venous drainage and venous ectasias. The goals of therapy should be tailored to individual patients and may include relief from symptoms or complete occlusion of a dAVF. The efficacy and safety of the treatment must be considered in conjunction with patient presentation and prognosis.

Carotid-Jugular Compression

Patients with Djindjian type I transverse or sigmoid sinus dAVFs or with fistulas of the cavernous sinus and otherwise normal ophthalmologic examinations may be treated conservatively. Intermittent manual compression of the carotid artery may be effective in eliminating dAVFs involving the ipsilateral cavernous sinus in patients with mild findings and no evidence of carotid vascular disease or other contraindications to carotid compression.[1] The ipsilateral carotid artery is compressed, using the contralateral hand, for approximately 5 minutes every waking hour for 1 to 3 days. If this is tolerated, the compression time is increased to 10 to 15 minutes of compression per waking hour. The compression, if properly performed, produces concomitant partial obstruction of the ipsilateral carotid artery and jugular vein. This results in the transient reduction of arteriovenous shunting by decreasing arterial inflow while simultaneously increasing the outlet venous pressure, thereby promoting spontaneous thrombosis within the nidus.

Embolization

The development of improved superselective angiographic catheter systems and embolic agents has increased the role of interventional neuroradiology in the management of dural AVMs, both primarily and preoperatively. Two strategies, transvenous and transarterial, are used, and their appropriate selection depends on the location and complexity of a dAVF, its vascular features, and the potential complications inherent to each technique.

Transvenous embolization with metallic coils or detachable balloons has been advocated primarily for the treatment of dAVFs involving the transverse, sigmoid, or cavernous sinuses. The technique involves a transfemoral or intraoperative approach to the affected venous sinus, following which the venous apparatus draining the fistula is occluded with coils, balloons, or liquid embolic agents (see **Figs. 1 and 2**). Several features are critical in appropriate patient selection for this method of treatment. (1) The segment of sinus to be occluded must be in proximity to the fistula and receive its entire venous drainage. (2) The sinus to be occluded should not be essential to the normal venous drainage of the brain. In this connection, the cerebral venous drainage must be thoroughly evaluated before embolization to determine the potential alternate pathways for cerebral venous outflow. (3) The target sinus must be completely occluded throughout the involved segment to avoid diversion of the fistula's drainage into confluent cerebral veins after embolization by way of a trapped sinus segment. Such redirection of a high-flow shunt into previously uninvolved low-capacitance venous channels may precipitate an acute venous infarct or hemorrhage.

Levrier and colleagues[18] developed a novel way to treat dAVFs that would preserve the venous sinus. In 10 patients, with fistulas from grade I to IV both with and without sinus stenosis, the researchers used a transvenous approach to angioplasty the involved sinus and then placed a self-expanding stent. Their follow-up at 7 months by conventional angiography revealed that four patients had complete dAVF occlusion and four had significantly reduced flow through the fistula. Two subjects refused repeat angiography. At 2 years, CT angiography confirmed stent patency in eight out of nine patients imaged.

Although usually safe and effective for the treatment of advanced sinus dAVFs, transvenous embolization reportedly is rarely associated with the development of de novo dAVFs at secondary intracranial sites after occlusion of the primary lesion. Although the cause of these secondary de novo fistulas is unclear, they may arise from angiogenesis induced by venous hypertension secondary to the occlusion of the major dural sinuses targeted by transvenous embolization.

Under some circumstances, transarterial embolization with liquid embolic agents offers advantages compared with a transvenous approach. Not infrequently, transvenous access to a dAVF is limited by venous sinus occlusion or high-grade stenoses preventing transvenous catheterization. Likewise, high-grade lesions emptying directly into remote cerebral veins may be inaccessible to uncomplicated venous catheterization. Fundamentally, however, transarterial delivery of a liquid embolic agent capable of permeating the vascular apparatus of the shunt provides the means for discrete definitive occlusion of a fistula site, reducing the likelihood for diversion of shunt flow into more dangerous alternate venous pathways and enabling closure of the fistula without necessarily sacrificing an entire venous conduit that may be critical to the drainage of normal brain parenchyma. Conversely, incomplete occlusion of a fistula by transarterial embolization is usually complicated by collateral reconstitution of the shunt through an increasingly complex angioarchitecture, potentially confounding further endovascular treatment.

The transarterial technique requires selective catheterization of individual feeding vessels (followed by superselective angiography to evaluate the vascular supply to the fistula, particularly with respect to potential anastomoses with the orbit or cerebral vasculature). Such anastomoses may not be demonstrable on the initial angiograms; however, they may become manifest as progressive embolization produces alterations in flow within the target vascular territory.

Guide wire–directed microcatheters are typically used in the catheterization of meningeal branches supplying such lesions. The embolic agents commonly used in transarterial embolization of dAVFs are liquid cyanoacrylate (NBCA), Onyx, polyvinyl alcohol foam (PVA), or ethanol. Ideally, liquid embolic agents, delivered close to the shunt under wedged microcatheter-induced flow arrest, present the best opportunity for embolotherapeutic cure of the lesion as they enable permeation of the collateral complex supplying a fistula and its immediate venous receptacle, thus permanently occluding the shunt. Such a degree of permeation is not possible using particulate agents that characteristically lodge within arterioles of the perifistula microcollateral network at a point proximal to the shunt. If not fully permeated, these microcollateral networks then evolve and re-establish flow through the shunt complex.

Nevertheless, PVA may find use in several situations. First, the initial use of PVA in embolizing the less favorable arterial supplies to a multipedicle fistula may facilitate more complete subsequent embolization of the shunt with liquid embolics through a safer conduit. The embolization of competing supplies to the shunt with PVA in this application permits the undiluted permeation of a fistula by the liquid embolic agent without fragmentation of the liquid stream. PVA also may be useful in reducing flow through low-velocity shunts, thereby facilitating thrombosis in these dAVFs. This can be particularly applicable in managing low-flow CSdAVFs and may be combined with manual compression in treating lesions also supplied by cavernous segment dural branches of the ipsilateral ICA.

In certain situations, partial embolization of dural fistulas may be performed in an attempt to ameliorate symptoms. For example, partial embolization of a CSdAVF can reduce intraocular pressure in patients suffering acute deterioration of visual acuity. Partial embolization also may be advocated in patients presenting with new-onset dementia or in those patients with severe tinnitus. Lastly, PVA and liquid embolic agents are used in the preoperative devascularization of dural fistulas proceeding to surgical excision. In this situation, particulate embolic agents, because of their low morbidity, are generally preferred and should be applied 1 to 2 days before surgery.

Over the past several years, Onyx has been increasingly used in the transarterial embolization of dAVFs, with various groups publishing results on larger cohorts of patients. Cognard and colleagues[19] enrolled 30 patients in a prospective trial: 10 were graded type II, 8 type III, and 12 type IV fistulas. They reported complete anatomic cure in 24 of 30 patients with only two complications, including a temporary cranial nerve palsy and postprocedure hemorrhage secondary to venous outlet thrombosis. Lv and colleagues[9,20] report their experience with 40 patients suffering from dAVFs. They report a complete occlusion rate of 25 of 40 (62.3%) patients from a total of 40. Nine patients suffered complications, including reflexive bradyarrhythmia in three patients, hemifacial hypoesthesia in three, hemifacial palsy in two, posterior infarction in two, jaw pain in one, hallucinations in one, Onyx migration in one, and retention of a microcatheter tip in one.

A few investigators have used Onyx in a transvenous approach to carotid-cavernous fistulas. After an unsuccessful embolization of a carotid-cavernous fistula using detachable coils and liquid adhesion agents, Arat and colleagues[21,22] successfully completed the embolization by injecting Onyx into the cavernous sinus forming a cast of the structure. Similarly, He and colleagues[23] report their experience in six patients using a combination of detachable coils and Onyx via a transvenous approach. Four of the six cases were completely embolized in a single attempt, whereas the other two required staged procedures. In these latter two cases, the patients suffered minor transient cranial nerve palsies. Suzuki and colleagues[24] report equally good results in three patients with spontaneous carotid-cavernous fistulas. In all these studies, patients experienced rapid relief of their neuro-ophthalmologic symptoms.

SUMMARY

Recent advances in endovascular therapies and studies of the anatomic and functional properties of dAVF led to a rapid evolution in their diagnosis and management. The decision of which approach and embolic agent to use for treatment of a dAVF must be tailored to individual cases, recognizing that the most effective approach for permanent dAVF treatment, particularly in high-flow shunts, may require a combination of approaches and embolic agents.

REFERENCES

1. Winn HR. Youmans neurological surgery edition: text with continually updated online. 2003.
2. Berenstein A, Lasjaunias P, Ter Brugge KG. Surgical neuroangiography. vol. 2, Clinical and endovascular treatment. 2nd edition. Springer; 2004.
3. Katsaridis V. Treatment of dural arteriovenous fistulas. Curr Treat Options Neurol 2009;11:35–40.
4. Geibprasert S, Pereira V, Krings T, et al. Dural arteriovenous shunts: a new classification of craniospinal epidural venous anatomical bases and clinical correlations. Stroke 2008;39:2783–94.
5. Cohen SD, Goins JL, Butler SG, et al. Dural arteriovenous fistula: diagnosis, treatment, and outcomes. Laryngoscope 2009;119:293–7.
6. Lasjaunias P, Halimi P, Lopez-Ibor L, et al. [Endovascular treatment of pure spontaneous dural vascular malformations. Review of 23 cases studied and treated between May 1980 and October 1983]. Neurochirurgie 1984;30:207–23 [in French].
7. Geibprasert S, Pereira V, Krings T, et al. Hydrocephalus in unruptured brain arteriovenous malformations: pathomechanical considerations, therapeutic implications, and clinical course. J Neurosurg 2009;110:500–7.
8. Zhou LF, Chen L, Song DL, et al. [Diagnosis and treatment of tentorial dural arteriovenous fistulae]. Zhonghua Wai Ke Za Zhi 2005;43:323–6 [in Chinese].
9. Lv X, Li Y, Wu Z. Endovascular treatment of anterior cranial fossa dural arteriovenous fistula. Neuroradiology 2008;50:433–7.
10. Akiba H, Tamakawa M, Hyodoh H, et al. Assessment of dural arteriovenous fistulas of the cavernous sinuses on 3D dynamic MR angiography. AJNR Am J Neuroradiol 2008;29:1652–7.
11. Bink A, Berkefeld J, Lüchtenberg M, et al. Coil embolization of cavernous sinus in patients with direct and dural arteriovenous fistula. Eur Radiol 2009;19:1443–9.
12. Stiebel-Kalish H, Setton A, Nimii Y, et al. Cavernous sinus dural arteriovenous malformations: patterns of venous drainage are related to clinical signs and symptoms. Ophthalmology 2002;109:1685–91.
13. Stiebel-Kalish H, Setton A, Berenstein A, et al. Bilateral orbital signs predict cortical venous drainage in cavernous sinus dural AVMs. Neurology 2002;58:1521–4.
14. Heidenreich JO, Schilling AM, Unterharnscheidt F, et al. Assessment of 3D-TOF-MRA at 3.0 Tesla in the characterization of the angioarchitecture of cerebral arteriovenous malformations: a preliminary study. (Stockholm, Sweden: 1987). Acta Radiol 2007;48:678–86.
15. Unlu E, Temizoz O, Albayram S, et al. Contrast-enhanced MR 3D angiography in the assessment of brain AVMs. Eur J Radiol 2006;60:367–78.
16. McGee KP, Ivanovic V, Felmlee JP, et al. MR angiography fusion technique for treatment planning of intracranial arteriovenous malformations. J Magn Reson Imaging 2006;23:361–9.
17. Meckel S, Maier M, Ruiz DS, et al. MR angiography of dural arteriovenous fistulas: diagnosis and follow-up after treatment using a time-resolved 3D contrast-enhanced technique. AJNR Am J Neuroradiol 2007;28:877–84.
18. Levrier O, Métellus P, Fuentes S, et al. Use of a self-expanding stent with balloon angioplasty in the treatment of dural arteriovenous fistulas involving the transverse and/or sigmoid sinus: functional and neuroimaging-based outcome in 10 patients. J Neurosurg 2006;104:254–63.
19. Cognard C, Januel AC, Silva NA, et al. Endovascular treatment of intracranial dural arteriovenous fistulas with cortical venous drainage: new management using Onyx. AJNR Am J Neuroradiol 2008;29:235–41.
20. Lv X, Li Y, Jiang C, et al. Endovascular treatment of brain arteriovenous fistulas. AJNR Am J Neuroradiol 2009;30:851–6.
21. Arat A, Cil BE, Vargel I, et al. Embolization of high-flow craniofacial vascular malformations with onyx. AJNR Am J Neuroradiol 2007;28:1409–14.
22. Arat A, Inci S. Treatment of a superior sagittal sinus dural arteriovenous fistula with Onyx: technical case report. Neurosurgery 2006;59:ONSE169–70 [discussion: ONSE169–70].
23. He HW, Jiang CH, Wu ZX, et al. Transvenous embolization with a combination of detachable coils and Onyx for a complicated cavernous dural arteriovenous fistula. Chin Med J 2008;121:1651–5.
24. Suzuki S, Lee DW, Jahan R, et al. Transvenous treatment of spontaneous dural carotid-cavernous fistulas using a combination of detachable coils and Onyx. AJNR Am J Neuroradiol 2006;27:1346–9.

Neuroendovascular Management of Vasospasm Following Aneurysmal Subarachnoid Hemorrhage

Pascal M. Jabbour, MD*, Stavropoula I. Tjoumakaris, MD,
Robert H. Rosenwasser, MD, FACS, FAHA

KEYWORDS

- Subarachnoid hemorrhage • Vasospasm
- Balloon angioplasty

Vasospasm affects 60% to 70% of patients after SAH, resulting in symptomatic ischemia in approximately half of those patients. It reaches maximal severity in the second week after SAH, typically resolving spontaneously in the third or fourth weeks. Vasospasm causes death or serious disability from infarction in up to one-third of patients with SAH. Delayed neurologic deterioration after SAH is presumed due to ischemic sequelae of vasospasm unless proven otherwise and attributed to other causes.

Although the pathogenesis is not clearly known, the risk is related to the amount of subarachnoid blood.[1–3]

The cause of cerebral vasospasm appears to be multifactorial, involving oxyhemoglobin, thromboxane, serotonin, and calcium.[4] Calcium activates calmodulin, which activates the myosin light-chain kinase and interacts with actin filaments to cause contractions blue.[5] Vessel tone is a balance between endothelium-derived constricting factors and endothelium-derived relaxation factors; nitric oxide is the most prominent in the latter. Studies have demonstrated that the dysfunction in vasospasm involve generally the vasodilator mechanisms. SAH lead to decreased nitric oxide activity.[6,7] Histologic analysis has shown morphologic changes of the spastic vessel wall, with necrosis and fibrosis of the intima and media.

Numerous advances in neurosurgical critical care, such as rheological manipulation of cerebral blood flow and the administration of calcium channel blockers, have reduced the ischemic and neurologic deficits associated with this devastating complication.

Although the treatment protocol of intravascular volume expansion, hemodilution, induced hypertension, and cardiac performance enhancement,[8–11] and the use of nimodipine,[12] have had a substantial beneficial effect on the treatment of this condition, it is not tolerated or is ineffective in some patients, who are subsequently susceptible to stroke, congestive heart failure, and death. Additional and alternative treatments for refractory vasospasm, particularly those specifically targeting the dilation of cerebral vessels, are needed.

Vasospasm may be monitored noninvasively by insonating the circle of Willis vessels and its branches using TCD. This noninvasive bedside procedure has a high sensitivity and specificity

Department of Neurological Surgery, Thomas Jefferson University, Jefferson Hospital for Neuroscience, 909 Walnut Street, 3rd Floor, Philadelphia, PA 19107, USA
* Corresponding author.
E-mail address: pascal.jabbour@jefferson.edu (P.M. Jabbour).

Neurosurg Clin N Am 20 (2009) 441–446
doi:10.1016/j.nec.2009.07.006

for vasospasm, but requires technical expertise and experience.[13] The course of TCD-documented vasospasm correlates closely with the course and clinical sequelae of vasospasm detected on angiography, and its severity closely reflects clinical sequelae of brain ischemia. Angiography may be used to confirm vasospasm in clinical situations where the cause of delayed neurologic deterioration is questionable, where TCD findings are nonconcordant with clinical progress, or where endovascular therapy for vasospasm is being contemplated.

ENDOVASCULAR OPTIONS

Cases of worsening vasospasm despite hyperdynamic therapy are considered for endovascular treatment.[14–18] The precise threshold for endovascular interventions remains controversial, with some centers advocating early and frequent endovascular treatment of spasm, while other centers reserve endovascular intervention for cases where symptomatic vasospasm does not respond to hyperdynamic therapy. It is clear that not all cases of severe TCD spasm will require endovascular intervention, and such therapy introduces an added risk, which must be considered and weighed. Conversely, endovascular treatment of spasm should not be delayed until actual infarction has developed.

Balloon Angioplasty

In 1984, the first reported use of angioplasty for the treatment of vasospasm was published by Zubkov and colleagues.[19] This opened up a new modality of treatment for patients who were medically refractory to reversal of their ischemic neurologic syndrome.[14,20,21] Despite successful improvement in the narrowing of the cerebral vessels with restored normal circulation time (as demonstrated angiographically), there have been many reports of equivocal clinical improvement.[14,16,22–24] It is possible that when patients are treated too late, there may be "end organ failure," despite restoration of blood flow, which is analogous to the thrombolysis theme and the restoration of blood flow to ischemic neural tissue after a thrombotic or embolic event.

Endovascular treatment of spasm traditionally has consisted of balloon angioplasty, mostly for large vessel spasm, or intraarterial pharmacologic infusions for more distal branch vasospasm. Angioplasty is associated with greater risk of arterial rupture or dissection, especially if applied to more distal vessels, but its effect is more durable than intraarterial pharmacologic infusions.[25–28] For patients with delayed SAH who have severe vasospasm proximal to the aneurysm site, a combined endovascular treatment with angioplasty and endovascular aneurysm coiling is safer than surgical clipping.[29,30]

The clinical success rate of TBA is variable.[18,22,23,31,32] The angiographic improvement with TBA seems to vary between 80% and 100% in most series. Clinical improvement ranges from 30% to 80%. Early treatment seems to be associated with better results.

There is a lack of randomized clinical studies that assess the effect of TBA on outcome, nor is much known of the long-term effects of TBA. The effect of angioplasty in the setting of cerebral vasospasm has been found to be lasting. Furthermore, the angioplastied vessels normalize in luminal diameter over time based on follow-up angiography. There are risks associated with this procedure including vessel perforation, unprotected aneurysm rerupture, branch occlusion, hemorrhagic infarction, and arterial dissection. Vessel rupture is reported in 4% of cases, usually with catastrophic outcome, and rebleeding from unclipped aneurysms is found in roughly 5% of cases.[21–23,33]

TIMING OF THE ANGIOPLASTY

Rosenwasser and colleagues,[18] studied the importance of the timing of the angioplasty. Between July 1993 and December 1997, a total of 466 patients were admitted to Thomas Jefferson University Hospital–Wills Neurosensory Institute with the diagnosis of "acute" aneurysmal subarachnoid hemorrhage. In the intensive care unit, all patients were treated prophylactically for hypervolemia and hemodilution, and induced hypertension, when, as shown by transcranial Doppler imaging, their velocities became elevated or showed a trend toward elevation with increasing ratios.[28,34,35] If the patients developed a new focal deficit or a change in their mental status, a computed tomographic scan was performed to eliminate a diagnosis of hydrocephalus or subsequent bleeding. Hypertensive, hypervolemic, hemodilution therapy would then be maximized to the point of elevating the mean arterial pressure to 130 to 140 mm Hg. If the patients did not demonstrate neurologic reversal within 60 minutes, they were transferred to the endovascular suite for angiography and possible angioplasty. All patients who required angioplasty received a ventriculostomy if one was not already in place **Fig. 1**.

Of the entire group of 466 patients, 93 (22%) underwent endovascular management of medically refractory cerebral vasospasm. Eighty-four

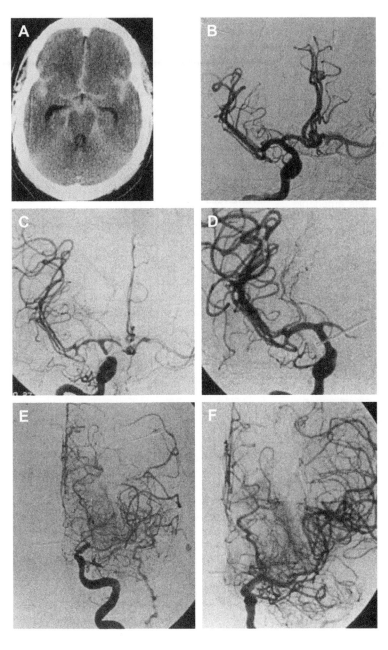

Fig. 1. (*A*) Noncontrast computed tomographic scan showing diffuse subarachnoid hemorrhage, Fisher's Grade 3, with early hydrocephalus as evidenced by enlarged temporal horns. (*B*) Right internal carotid angiogram demonstrating no spasm and a small anterior communicating artery aneurysm. (*C*) Right internal carotid angiogram 1 week postoperatively demonstrating severe spasm of the right internal carotid system. (*D*) Angiogram, posttreatment. (*E*) Left internal carotid angiogram demonstrating severe spasm of the supraclinoid carotid and middle cerebral artery, pretreatment. (*F*) Left internal carotid angiogram, posttreatment.

of these patients were available for a minimum of 6 months of follow-up. The breakdown of these 84 patients by grade was as follows: Grade I, 2 of 33 patients (6%), Grade II, 9 of 84 patients (10%), Grade III, 57 of 260 patients (22%), and Grade IV, 16 of 42 patients (38%). Fifty-one patients (61%) underwent endovascular management within a 2-hour window because of the inability to reverse the patients' neurologic deficits with medical measures. In this group, 90% of patients demonstrated improvement angiographically and 70% of patients sustained clinical improvement, based on Glasgow Coma Scale parameters as previously outlined ($P<.01$) ([chi]^2 = 8.02). Thirty-three patients (39%) failed to improve with the best medical therapy available; they were treated in more than a 2-hour window (range: 2 hours, 15 minutes–17 hours) and had 88% angiographic improvement, but only 40% sustained clinical improvement. Clinical improvement was noted as early as 60 minutes after the procedure when gross motor movement could be evaluated. However, global improvement (Glasgow Coma Scale) continued for up to 48 hours, and further recovery continued during the hospital stay.

TECHNIQUE

The protocol involves transfemoral angiography with placement of an 8-French femoral sheath. Full heparinization is performed to achieve an activated clotting time of twice baseline, to prevent thromboembolic complications and all of these patients received general anesthesia and had neurophysiological monitoring while being treated. Endovascular management is performed using an Endeavor silicone balloon with inflations with thumb pressure for periods of 1 to 5 seconds or a stealth system (Target Therapeutics, Boston Scientific, Boston, MA, USA). Vessels amenable to angioplasty include all the intracranial proximal vessels: ICA, M1, A1, P1, Vertebrals, and Basilar. For more distal vasospasm, intraarterial pharmacologic infusion should be considered because trying to perform an angioplasty on more distal vessels carries a higher risk of rupturing the vessel.

Intraarterial Infusion

Recently, a variety of calcium channel antagonists and other vasodilators have been studied using intrathecal and intraarterial delivery. Intrathecal nitroprusside has been proven safe, but efficacy is still controversial.[36–38] The use of intraarterial calcium channel blockers such as nicardipine, verapamil, or nimodipine has been shown to significantly reduce TCD velocities, to provide clinical improvement in up to 72% of patients, and to increase vessel caliber by 44%.[39–41] The application of nicardipine prolonged-release implants in the basal cistern of Fisher Grade III SAH patients has shown promising results.[42] Future therapies for vasospasm will be aimed at improved delivery systems and developing biologic agents that target the numerous cellular substrates responsible for vasospasm. Many animal research studies are being performed on intrathecal immunotherapy, another vast field to explore.[43–45]

SUMMARY

Neurosurgical critical care has made dramatic improvements in the perioperative management of the patient suffering from aneurysmal subarachnoid hemorrhage. Calcium channel blockers and hypervolemic hemodilution therapy continue to be a cornerstone in the management of this problem and are effective in approximately 80% of patients.

There are patients who are refractory to medical therapy; angioplasty in the affected territory may be of benefit in improving not only the angiographic appearance but also the ultimate outcome for the patient, if performed in a timely fashion. The authors' experience indicates that a 2-hour window may exist for the restoration of blood flow, which is analogous to a patient who presents with a vascular-related event from either an embolic or thrombotic occlusion. The authors concur with other investigators that, although these results are encouraging, randomized controlled trials in a prospective fashion are necessary to determine the true efficacy of angioplasty in the treatment of vasospasm and whether it influences ultimate outcome.

REFERENCES

1. Fisher M, Cameron DG. Concerning cerebral vasospasm. Neurology 1953;3:468.
2. Friedman JA, Goerss SJ, Meyer FB, et al. Volumetric quantification of Fisher Grade 3 aneurysmal subarachnoid hemorrhage: a novel method to predict symptomatic vasospasm on admission computerized tomography scans. J Neurosurg 2002;97:401.
3. Suzuki H, Muramatsu M, Kojima T, et al. Intracranial heme metabolism and cerebral vasospasm after aneurysmal subarachnoid hemorrhage. Stroke 2003;34:2796.
4. Sonobe M, Suzuki J. Vasospasmogenic substance produced following subarachnoid haemorrhage, and its fate. Acta Neurochir (Wien) 1978;44:97.
5. Winder SJ, Allen BG, Clement-Chomienne O, et al. Regulation of smooth muscle actin-myosin interaction and force by calponin. Acta Physiol Scand 1998;164:415.
6. Inagawa T. Cerebral vasospasm in elderly patients treated by early operation for ruptured intracranial aneurysms. Acta Neurochir (Wien) 1992;115:79.
7. Sobey CG. Cerebrovascular dysfunction after subarachnoid haemorrhage: novel mechanisms and directions for therapy. Clin Exp Pharmacol Physiol 2001;28:926.
8. Kassell NF, Peerless SJ, Durward QJ, et al. Treatment of ischemic deficits from vasospasm with intravascular volume expansion and induced arterial hypertension. Neurosurgery 1982;11:337.
9. Kosnik EJ, Hunt WE. Postoperative hypertension in the management of patients with intracranial arterial aneurysms. J Neurosurg 1976;45:148.
10. Pritz MB, Giannotta SL, Kindt GW, et al. Treatment of patients with neurological deficits associated with cerebral vasospasm by intravascular volume expansion. Neurosurgery 1978;3:364.
11. Wood JH, Simeone FA, Fink EA, et al. Hypervolemic hemodilution in experimental focal cerebral ischemia. Elevation of cardiac output, regional cortical blood flow, and ICP after intravascular volume expansion with low molecular weight dextran. J Neurosurg 1983;59:500.

12. Allen GS, Ahn HS, Preziosi TJ, et al. Cerebral arterial spasm—a controlled trial of nimodipine in patients with subarachnoid hemorrhage. N Engl J Med 1983;308:619.

13. Kim P, Schini VB, Sundt TM Jr, et al. Reduced production of cGMP underlies the loss of endothelium-dependent relaxations in the canine basilar artery after subarachnoid hemorrhage. Circ Res 1992;70:248.

14. Eskridge JM, McAuliffe W, Song JK, et al. Balloon angioplasty for the treatment of vasospasm: results of first 50 cases. Neurosurgery 1998;42:510.

15. Eskridge JM, Newell DW, Pendleton GA. Transluminal angioplasty for treatment of vasospasm. Neurosurg Clin N Am 1990;1:387.

16. Higashida RT, Halbach VV, Cahan LD, et al. Transluminal angioplasty for treatment of intracranial arterial vasospasm. J Neurosurg 1989;71:648.

17. Rosenwasser RH. Endovascular tools for the neurosurgeon. Clin Neurosurg 2002;49:115.

18. Rosenwasser RH, Armonda RA, Thomas JE, et al. Therapeutic modalities for the management of cerebral vasospasm: timing of endovascular options. Neurosurgery 1999;44:975.

19. Zubkov YN, Nikiforov BM, Shustin VA. Balloon catheter technique for dilatation of constricted cerebral arteries after aneurysmal SAH. Acta Neurochir (Wien) 1984;70:65.

20. Eskridge JM. Interventional neuroradiology. Radiology 1989;172:991.

21. Eskridge JM, Song JK. A practical approach to the treatment of vasospasm. AJNR Am J Neuroradiol 1997;18:1653.

22. Bejjani GK, Bank WO, Olan WJ, et al. The efficacy and safety of angioplasty for cerebral vasospasm after subarachnoid hemorrhage. Neurosurgery 1998;42:979.

23. Polin RS, Coenen VA, Hansen CA, et al. Efficacy of transluminal angioplasty for the management of symptomatic cerebral vasospasm following aneurysmal subarachnoid hemorrhage. J Neurosurg 2000;92:284.

24. Yamamoto Y, Smith RR, Bernanke DH. Mechanism of action of balloon angioplasty in cerebral vasospasm. Neurosurgery 1992;30:1.

25. Elliott JP, Newell DW, Lam DJ, et al. Comparison of balloon angioplasty and papaverine infusion for the treatment of vasospasm following aneurysmal subarachnoid hemorrhage. J Neurosurg 1998;88:277.

26. Kassell NF, Helm G, Simmons N, et al. Treatment of cerebral vasospasm with intra-arterial papaverine. J Neurosurg 1992;77:848.

27. Linskey ME, Horton JA, Rao GR, et al. Fatal rupture of the intracranial carotid artery during transluminal angioplasty for vasospasm induced by subarachnoid hemorrhage. Case report. J Neurosurg 1991; 74:985.

28. Newell DW, Eskridge JM, Mayberg MR, et al. Angioplasty for the treatment of symptomatic vasospasm following subarachnoid hemorrhage. J Neurosurg 1989;71:654.

29. Brisman JL, Roonprapunt C, Song JK, et al. Intentional partial coil occlusion followed by delayed clip application to wide-necked middle cerebral artery aneurysms in patients presenting with severe vasospasm. Report of two cases. J Neurosurg 2004;101:154.

30. Murayama Y, Song JK, Uda K, et al. Combined endovascular treatment for both intracranial aneurysm and symptomatic vasospasm. AJNR Am J Neuroradiol 2003;24:133.

31. Higashida RT, Halbach VV, Dowd CF, et al. Intravascular balloon dilatation therapy for intracranial arterial vasospasm: patient selection, technique, and clinical results. Neurosurg Rev 1992;15:89.

32. Newell DW, Eskridge JM, Aaslid R. Current indications and results of cerebral angioplasty. Acta Neurochir Suppl 2001;77:181.

33. Eskridge JM, Newell DW, Winn HR. Endovascular treatment of vasospasm. Neurosurg Clin N Am 1994;5:437.

34. Grosset DG, Straiton J, du Trevou M, et al. Prediction of symptomatic vasospasm after subarachnoid hemorrhage by rapidly increasing transcranial Doppler velocity and cerebral blood flow changes. Stroke 1992;23:674.

35. Newell DW, Winn HR. Transcranial Doppler in cerebral vasospasm. Neurosurg Clin N Am 1990;1:319.

36. Rosenwasser RH. Re: Safety of intraventricular sodium nitroprusside and thiosulfate for the treatment of cerebral vasospasm in the intensive care unit setting. Stroke 2002;33:1165.

37. Thomas JE, Rosenwasser RH. Reversal of severe cerebral vasospasm in three patients after aneurysmal subarachnoid hemorrhage: initial observations regarding the use of intraventricular sodium nitroprusside in humans. Neurosurgery 1999;44:48.

38. Thomas JE, Rosenwasser RH, Armonda RA, et al. Safety of intrathecal sodium nitroprusside for the treatment and prevention of refractory cerebral vasospasm and ischemia in humans. Stroke 1999; 30:1409.

39. Badjatia N, Topcuoglu MA, Pryor JC, et al. Preliminary experience with intra-arterial nicardipine as a treatment for cerebral vasospasm. AJNR Am J Neuroradiol 2004;25:819.

40. Biondi A, Ricciardi GK, Puybasset L, et al. Intra-arterial nimodipine for the treatment of symptomatic cerebral vasospasm after aneurysmal subarachnoid hemorrhage: preliminary results. AJNR Am J Neuroradiol 2004;25:1067.

41. Feng L, Fitzsimmons BF, Young WL, et al. Intraarterially administered verapamil as adjunct therapy for cerebral vasospasm: safety and 2-year experience. AJNR Am J Neuroradiol 2002;23:1284.

42. Kasuya H, Onda H, Sasahara A, et al. Application of nicardipine prolonged-release implants: analysis of 97 consecutive patients with acute subarachnoid hemorrhage. Neurosurgery 2005;56:895.

43. Cirak B, Kiymaz N, Ari HH, et al. The effects of endothelin antagonist BQ-610 on cerebral vascular wall following experimental subarachnoid hemorrhage and cerebral vasospasm. Clin Auton Res 2004;14:197.

44. Frazier JL, Pradilla G, Wang PP, et al. Inhibition of cerebral vasospasm by intracranial delivery of ibuprofen from a controlled-release polymer in a rabbit model of subarachnoid hemorrhage. J Neurosurg 2004;101:93.

45. Pradilla G, Wang PP, Legnani FG, et al. Prevention of vasospasm by anti-CD11/CD18 monoclonal antibody therapy following subarachnoid hemorrhage in rabbits. J Neurosurg 2004;101:88.

Neuroendovascular Management of Carotid Cavernous Fistulae

Stavropoula I. Tjoumakaris, MD*, Pascal M. Jabbour, MD,
Robert H. Rosenwasser, MD, FACS, FAHA

KEYWORDS

- Carotid cavernous fistula • Management
- Endovascular • Arteriovenous fistula • Direct • Indirect

Carotid-cavernous fistulae (CCFs) are an abnormal communication between arteries and veins located in the cavernous sinus. The term *pulsatile exophthalmos* describes previous attempts to characterize this vascular disorder dating back to 1809.[1] The constellation of symptoms in this disease is related to increased pressure within the cavernous sinus. Treatment options vary from conservative manual carotid compression to microsurgical and endovascular approaches. Current advances in endovascular techniques have revolutionized the treatment of CCF and now provide a safe and efficacious therapeutic option.

CLASSIFICATION AND ETIOLOGY

Several classification schemes have described CCFs based on their etiology (traumatic or spontaneous), flow rate (high or low), and communication with the internal carotid artery (ICA) (direct or indirect). The most widely accepted classification is that proposed by Barrow and colleagues,[2] which categorizes CCFs into four distinct types based on their arterial supply:

> Type A: direct communication of the fistula with the ICA
>
> Type B: CCF arterial supply provided by meningeal ICA branches
>
> Type C: CCF arterial supply provided by meningeal external carotid artery branches

> Type D: CCF arterial supply provided by meningeal branches of both the ICA and the external carotid artery

Type A is a direct CCF with a high flow rate (**Fig. 1**). The most common etiology of this type is traumatic disruption of the vessel wall. Such disruptions might stem from, for example, frontal blunt trauma, optic globe injury, gunshot wounds, and iatrogenic causes (following transphenoidal surgery or glycerol rhizotomy). These fistulae are less likely to resolve spontaneously and may require intervention if symptomatic. The remaining types are indirect and are best described as dural arteriovenous malformations (**Fig. 2**). Their rate of flow and exact etiology are variable. They have been associated with pregnancy, cavernous sinus thrombosis, sinusitis, and minor trauma.[3]

SYMPTOMS AND PATHOPHYSIOLOGY

The clinical presentation of CCF is a direct consequence of elevation in intracavernous pressure. This pressure is transmitted anteriorly to the ipsilateral orbit and posteriorly to the inferior petrosal sinus.[4] The elevated orbital venous pressure presents as the classic triad of exophthalmos, conjunctival chemosis, and cephalic bruit. In a CCF series by Venuela and colleagues,[5] the incidence of the first two symptoms was much higher than the last (90% vs 25%). Diplopia is another commonly reported symptom in CCF patients. The etiology is the proximity of cranial nerves III, IV, and VI in

Department of Neurological Surgery, Thomas Jefferson University Hospital, 909 Walnut Street, 3rd Floor, Philadelphia, PA 19107, USA
* Corresponding author.
E-mail address: stavropoula@gmail.com (S.I. Tjoumakaris).

Neurosurg Clin N Am 20 (2009) 447–452
doi:10.1016/j.nec.2009.07.013
1042-3680/09/$ – see front matter. Published by Elsevier Inc.

neurosurgery.theclinics.com

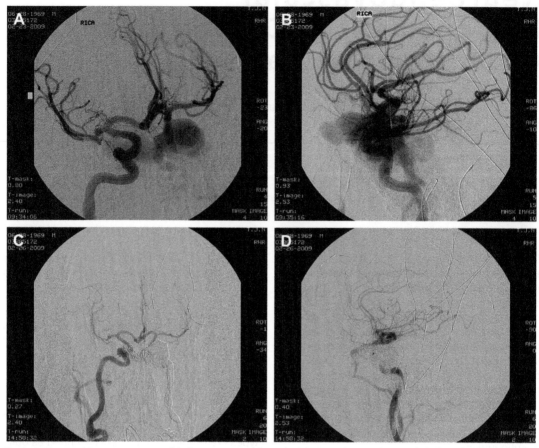

Fig. 1. Patient with acute onset of left proptosis, blurred vision, and complete ophthalmoplegia, following trauma. Frontal (*A*) and lateral (*B*) digital subtraction angiogram views of right ICA showing a large type I left CCF. Frontal (*C*) and lateral (*D*) midarterial phase angiogram views after right ICA injection and following fistula obliteration with platinum coils and left ICA deconstruction with Onyx. Filling of distal left ICA circulation is supplied from the contralateral circulation.

the cavernous sinus and the mechanical restriction of the extraocular muscles they supply. Visual loss is the most feared complication of retinal ischemia in CCFs. This is an ophthalmologic emergency and warrants immediate treatment. Epistaxis and intra-cranial hemorrhage are less frequently described symptoms related to increased venous pressure.[4] These symptoms usually have an acute onset in direct CCF and a chronic progression in the indirect types.

PRETHERAPEUTIC EVALUATION

The clinical diagnosis of CCF is not difficult. However, implementing the best therapeutic regimen requires careful medical, radiographic, and angiographic evaluation. As in any other angiographic therapy, careful evaluation of patient comorbidities, such as diabetes, hypertension, and athesclerotic disease and medical clearance,

should be obtained prior to intervention. Initial acquisition of a noncontrast head CT scan allows for careful examination of possible cranial injuries, such as bony fractures, intracranial hematomas, and sinus opacification. An MRI scan could provide soft tissue information, such as ophthalmic vein prominence, ocular muscle congestion, cortical vein congestion, and lateral bulging of the cavernous sinus.[6]

Cerebral angiography is crucial for the definitive diagnosis of CCF, classification, and planning of endovascular intervention. Femoral access contralateral to the site of pathology is obtained. Global cortical arterial circulation and venous drainage should be inspected for any abnormal findings. The cavernous portion of the ICA is imaged under high magnification. The exact location of the fistula and its relationship to the ICA are determined. Other associated vascular lesions, such as traumatic pseudoaneurysm, arterial

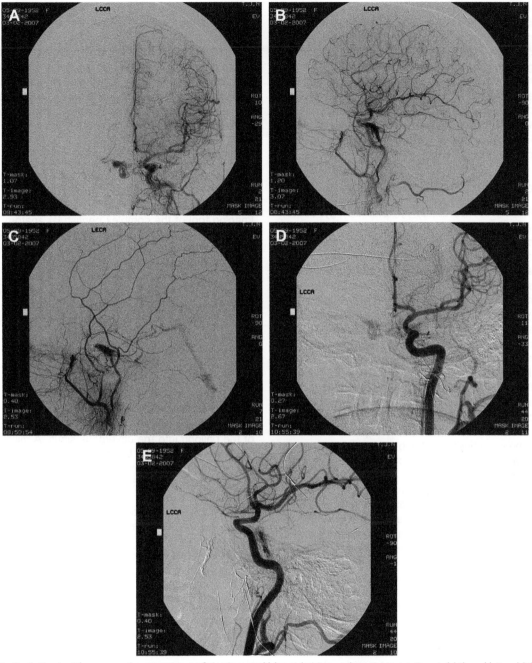

Fig. 2. Patient with progressive symptoms of tinnitus and blurred vision, subacute onset. Frontal (*A*) and lateral (*B*) digital subtraction angiogram views of left common carotid artery showing a type III left CCF. (*C*) Left external carotid artery injection, lateral midarterial phase, showing meningeal branch supply to the CCF. Frontal (*D*) and lateral (*E*) midarterial phase angiogram views of left common carotid artery, following Onyx embolization of feeding external carotid artery branches.

dissection, and venous thrombosis, are noted. Examination of the rate of arterial flow at the CCF in relation to global cerebral blood flow may reveal an arterial steal, which usually affects the ophthalmic artery territory.[6] Finally, the venous drainage of the fistula should be examined for presence of subarachnoid venous reflux, associated venous plexus or ectasia, and sinus thrombosis.

High-flow CCFs may be difficult to capture in digital subtraction angiography, even on selective high frame rates. Certain maneuvers can be implemented to slow the fistula flow and facilitate image capture. The Mehringer-Hieshima maneuver entails compression of the ipsilateral common carotid artery during slow-rate angiographic imaging of the ipsilateral ICA. The Huber maneuver also involves compression of the ipsilateral common carotid artery. However, the maneuver must be performed during ipsilateral vertebral artery injection. This technique allows for slower imaging of the CCF through a posterior communicating artery, if present.[7]

CURRENT TREATMENT

In the presence of mild symptomatology, conservative management with careful follow-up of intraocular pressures, visual acuity, and cranial neuropathies should be implemented. This is established with digital compression of the ipsilateral carotid artery and jugular vein. Compression must be performed while the patient is sitting or lying down with the contralateral hand. The latter ensures that if ischemia and weakness develop, the symptomatic arm will fall away from the neck, thus allowing cortical revascularization. This treatment is usually ineffective in the high-flow CCFs, which usually require endovascular intervention. Contraindications to carotid-jugular compression are symptomatic bradycardia with carotid compression and significant cortical venous drainage.[8] Compression of the jugular vein could obstruct venous outflow, leading to elevated cerebral venous pressure and resulting in venous infarction or hemorrhage.

In symptomatic patients failing conservative therapy and in clinical emergencies, the endovascular approach is the primary treatment option. Signs and symptoms that warrant immediate intervention are acute visual loss, epistaxis, sphenoid sinus aneurysm, and decreased mental status.[6] Microsurgical management of CCFs via skull-base frontotemporal cavernous sinus exposure is reserved for symptomatic patients who fail endovascular therapy.[4] Stereotactic radiosurgery is investigated in several institutions for the treatment of CCFs. Although preliminary data show that radiosurgery may be effective in the treatment of indirect CCFs, significant disadvantages exist, such as an average 8-month lag between treatment and effect, high recurrence rates, and inability to manage emergencies and traumatic fistulae.[9,10]

ENDOVASCULAR TECHNIQUES

Endovascular management of CCFs can be performed with several techniques. The goal of treatment is to obliterate the communication between the ICA and cavernous sinus, while maintaining patency of the former. The treatment options available include transarterial obliteration with detachable balloons, embolization material, and covered stents; transvenous embolization; and ICA sacrifice.[7] The treatment choice is individualized based on the exact anatomy of the fistula, the type and size of the arterial defect, and operator's preference.

Detachable Balloons

Transarterial balloon detachment is the endovascular treatment of choice for direct CCF.[11–13] Three-dimensional angiography provides a useful imaging tool of the complex perifistular anatomy, facilitating successful balloon deployment.[14] The balloon is flow-directed through the fistula into the cavernous sinus. It is subsequently inflated with iso-osmolar contrast material to a size slightly larger than the fistula. This maneuver prevents prolapse of the balloon into the ICA. A single silicone balloon is usually sufficient for most CCFs. However, at times, multiple balloons may be required. Following successful balloon deployment, cerebral angiography is repeated to ensure closure of the fistula and patency of the ICA.

Successful fistula embolization with this technique may not always be possible. Complexity of the perifistular anatomy may prevent navigation of the balloon into the cavernous sinus. A microguidewire within the balloon may assist flow through the intricate turns of ICA and fistula. Inadequate embolization may occur with early balloon detachment, deflation, or rupture by contact with a bony fragment. Over time, the balloon may eventually deflate. Following deflation, creation of a venous pouch at the previous inflation site may occur. These spontaneously resolve in the majority of cases and rarely become symptomatic.[6]

Coil and Material Embolization

Transarterial CCF embolization can be performed with the same technique as aneurysmal embolization. A microcatheter is floated through the ICA tear into the cavernous sinus. Embolization can be achieved with platinum coils or liquid embolic agents (see **Fig. 1**).[15] Coil embolization may be stent-assisted in the case of a large ICA defect to prevent coil prolapse into the parent vessel.[16] Other embolization materials used are N-butyl-cyano-acrylate (NBCA), such as Trufill NBCA (Cordis Neurovascular, Miami, FL); ethylene-vinyl alcohol copolymer (EVOC), such as Onyx (ev3 Neurovascular, Irvine, CA) (see **Fig. 2**), and silk.[7]

The technical difficulties of this technique are related to the presence of multiple small ICA feeders into the cavernous sinus, which makes catheterization extremely challenging. Staging of this approach may allow for long-term fistula obliteration. The main risks of this technique are the embolization of thrombus material in the distal circulation and occlusion of the ICA.

Transvenous Embolization

Transvenous embolization is the preferred treatment for indirect CCFs.[13] It can be performed via a posterior or anterior route. The posterior route from the common femoral vein to the internal jugular vein, the inferior petrosal sinus, and into the cavernous sinus is most commonly used. Alternatively, an anterior approach may be followed from the superior ophthalmic vein via the facial vein. Less commonly used transvenous approaches are through the lateral pterygoid plexus, superior petrosal sinus, cortical veins, and the inferior ophthalmic vein.[7,17–19] Once the cavernous sinus is catheterized, embolization similar to that with the transarterial approach is performed. Coils, NBCA, and Onyx have been successfully used in this technique.

The advantages of this method are the ability to cure the fistula in a single session, its simplicity compared to the transarterial method, and higher long-term success rates.[7] Its use in the acute fistula stages may be hazardous because the venous walls have not acquired wall-thickening via arterialization.[6] Navigation through the venous system and mechanical perforation are technical challenges in this procedure. If the femoral vein route is inaccessible, then cut-down or direct stick may be performed.

Stent Embolization

The use of polyfluorotetraethylene- (PTFE-) or Gore-Tex–covered stents has been reported in the treatment of direct CCFs. Placement of this impermeable barrier across the ICA defect obliterates the fistula, while preserving ICA patency.[20–22] Studies on successful deployment of covered stents are limited and long-term follow-up results are lacking. Although their use is a promising endovascular technique, further data are required prior to their establishment as an acceptable method for treatment of CCFs.

Carotid Occlusion

Extensive vessel-wall injury to the ICA may result in direct CCFs that are not amenable to endovascular repair. In a life-saving emergency, arterial sacrifice may be required for the definitive treatment of such large fistulae (see **Fig. 1**). In less-urgent clinical scenarios, a temporary balloon occlusion testing is warranted to ensure distal perfusion from collateral circulation. Occlusion of the ipsilateral ICA is performed with coil embolization in a distal-to-proximal approach. This technique prevents retrograde arterial filling of the fistula from the supraclinoid ICA.[7] An alternative technique is fistula entrapment between two balloons, proximal and distal to the fistula, in close proximity to each other.[6]

TREATMENT OUTCOME

The long-term results for the endovascular treatment of CCFs are favorable with satisfactory angiographic follow-up. The success rate for closure of direct CCFs is reported as 82% to 99%, whereas that of indirect CCFs as 70% to 78%.[8,23–25] In a study by Higashida and colleagues,[25] 206 direct CCFs were treated via different endovascular approaches, with an angiographic occlusion rate of 99% and ICA patency rate of 88%. In a series of 89 patients with direct CCFs, Gupta and colleagues[26] treated 79 with detachable balloons and 10 with arterial coil-occlusion. In 1-month follow-up, the clinical cure rate was 89%, with 10% of patients experiencing significant improvement. The main complications reported were worsening oculomotor palsy and ipislateral ICA occlusion with an incidence of 10% to 40%.[8,23]

SUMMARY

Neuroendovascular intervention has emerged as the preferred treatment for direct and indirect carotid cavernous fistulae with favorable long-term outcomes. The endovascular approach is tailored to the type, anatomy, and extent of each fistula. Novel techniques, such as placement of stent grafts, have shown some promise in preliminary clinical studies.

REFERENCES

1. Locke CE. Intracranial arterio-venous aneurism or pulsating exophthalmos. Ann Surg 1924;80:1–24.
2. Barrow DL, Spector RH, Braun IF, et al. Classification and treatment of spontaneous carotid-cavernous sinus fistulas. J Neurosurg 1985;62:248–56.
3. Kwan E, Hieshima GB, Higashida RT, et al. Interventional neuroradiology in neuro-ophthalmology. J Clin Neuroophthalmol 1989;9:83–97.
4. Winn HR. Youmans neurological surgery edition: text with continually updated online. 2003.
5. Viñuela F, Fox AJ, Debrun GM, et al. Spontaneous carotid-cavernous fistulas: clinical, radiological, and therapeutic considerations. Experience with 20 cases. J Neurosurg 1984;60:976–84.

6. Berenstein A, Lasjaunias P, Ter Brugge KG. Surgical neuroangiography. vol. 2, Clinical and endovascular treatment. 2nd edition. Springer; 2004.

7. Gemmete JJ, Ansari SA, Gandhi DM. Endovascular techniques for treatment of carotid-cavernous fistula. J Neuroophthalmol 2009;29:62–71.

8. Halbach VV, Higashida RT, Hieshima GB, et al. Dural fistulas involving the cavernous sinus: results of treatment in 30 patients. Radiology 1987;163:437–42.

9. Pollock BE, Nichols DA, Garrity JA, et al. Stereotactic radiosurgery and particulate embolization for cavernous sinus dural arteriovenous fistulae. Neurosurgery 1999;45:459–66 [discussion: 466–57].

10. Barcia-Salorio JL, Soler F, Barcia JA, et al. Radiosurgery of carotid-cavernous fistulae. Acta Neurochir Suppl 1994;62:10–2.

11. Teng MM, Chang CY, Chiang JH, et al. Double-balloon technique for embolization of carotid cavernous fistulas. AJNR Am J Neuroradiol 2000; 21:1753–6.

12. Goto K, Hieshima GB, Higashida RT, et al. Treatment of direct carotid cavernous sinus fistulae. Various therapeutic approaches and results in 148 cases. Acta Radiol Suppl 1986;369:576–9.

13. Barnwell SL, O'Neill OR. Endovascular therapy of carotid cavernous fistulas. Neurosurg Clin N Am 1994;5:485–95.

14. Kwon BJ, Han MH, Kang HS, et al. Endovascular occlusion of direct carotid cavernous fistula with detachable balloons: usefulness of 3D angiography. Neuroradiology 2005;47:271–81.

15. Xie W, Shi J, Liu C, et al. [Endovascular treatment of carotid-cavernous sinus fistulae]. Zhonghua Wai Ke Za Zhi 1998;36:401–2 [in Chinese].

16. Morón FE, Klucznik RP, Mawad ME, et al. Endovascular treatment of high-flow carotid cavernous fistulas by stent-assisted coil placement. AJNR Am J Neuroradiol 2005;26:1399–404.

17. Gioulekas J, Mitchell P, Tress B, et al. Embolization of carotid cavernous fistulas via the superior ophthalmic vein. Aust N Z J Ophthalmol 1997;25:47–53.

18. Annesley-Williams DJ, Goddard AJ, Brennan RP, et al. Endovascular approach to treatment of indirect carotico-cavernous fistulae. Br J Neurosurg 2001; 15:228–33.

19. Théaudin M, Saint-Maurice JP, Chapot R, et al. Diagnosis and treatment of dural carotid-cavernous fistulas: a consecutive series of 27 patients. J Neurol Neurosurg Psychiatr 2007;78:174–9.

20. Archondakis E, Pero G, Valvassori L, et al. Angiographic follow-up of traumatic carotid cavernous fistulas treated with endovascular stent graft placement. AJNR Am J Neuroradiol 2007;28:342–7.

21. Gomez F, Escobar W, Gomez AM, et al. Treatment of carotid cavernous fistulas using covered stents: midterm results in seven patients. AJNR Am J Neuroradiol 2007;28:1762–8.

22. Madan A, Mujic A, Daniels K, et al. Traumatic carotid artery-cavernous sinus fistula treated with a covered stent. Report of two cases. J Neurosurg 2006;104: 969–73.

23. Lewis AI, Tomsick TA, Tew JM. Management of 100 consecutive direct carotid-cavernous fistulas: results of treatment with detachable balloons. Neurosurgery 1995;36:239–44 [discussion: 244–235].

24. Debrun G, Lacour P, Viñuela F, et al. Treatment of 54 traumatic carotid-cavernous fistulas. J Neurosurg 1981;55:678–92.

25. Higashida RT, Halbach VV, Tsai FY, et al. Interventional neurovascular treatment of traumatic carotid and vertebral artery lesions: results in 234 cases. AJR Am J Roentgenol 1989;153:577–82.

26. Gupta AK, Purkayastha S, Krishnamoorthy T, et al. Endovascular treatment of direct carotid cavernous fistulae: a pictorial review. Neuroradiology 2006;48: 831–9.

Neuroendovascular Management of Tumors and Vascular Malformations of the Head and Neck

Laligam N. Sekhar, MD, FACS[a,b,d],*, Arundhati Biswas, MD[a], Danial Hallam, MD[a,b], Louis J. Kim, MD[a,b], James Douglas, MD[c], Basavaraj Ghodke, MD[a,b]

KEYWORDS

- Embolization • Onyx • Brain arteriovenous malformation
- Dural AV fistulas • Tumors

Endovascular procedures are rapidly expanding as treatment options for cerebrovascular diseases and neoplasms of the head and neck and are becoming less invasive but more effective. There are potentially dangerous anastomoses between the extracranial and intracranial circulations; hence, thorough knowledge of the anatomy is essential to minimize the risk of cranial nerve palsies, blindness, or neurologic deficits. It is essential to understand the scientific basis of treatment rationale based on advancing new neuroimaging techniques to better serve patients. An interdisciplinary approach and treatment in high-volume centers are vital to obtain maximal benefit for patients.

Endovascular therapy has continuously evolved and improved since it was first described in 1904.[1] Rapid advances in the field have resulted in the ability to safely embolize and effectively treat craniocervical neoplasms and vascular malformations. Preoperative embolization of tumors reduces intraoperative blood loss, shortens surgical time, and decreases surgical morbidity.[2,3] This technique involves superselective catheterization of the feeding arteries to the tumor bed with infusion of embolic particles to saturate the tumor bed in the hopes of inducing necrosis. For some malignant head and neck tumors, selective infusion of chemotherapeutic agents has been performed as part of combined therapy.

The endovascular therapy of brain arteriovenous malformations (AVMs), dural arteriovenous fistulas (DAVFs), carotico-cavernous fistulas, and vein of Galen malformations is part of the therapeutic strategy. This article presents the indications, techniques, results, and potential complications of endovascular embolization of craniocervical vascular malformations, and craniocervical tumors.

BRAIN ARTERIOVENOUS MALFORMATIONS
Indications for Treatment

Embolization of an AVM is mainly used as an adjunct to surgical treatment to reduce the size of an AVM or make it safer for surgery, although in some patients with small AVMs and a few arterial feeders, "angiographic cure" of an AVM may

[a] Department of Neurosurgery, Harborview Medical Center, University of Washington, 325 9th Avenue, Box 359766, Seattle, WA 98105-9950, USA
[b] Department of Radiology, Harborview Medical Center, University of Washington, Seattle, WA, USA
[c] Department of Radiation Oncology, Harborview Medical Center, University of Washington, Seattle, WA, USA
[d] Department of Neurological Surgery, Harborview Medical Center, Box 359766, Seattle, WA 98104, USA
* Corresponding author. Department of Neurological Surgery, Harborview Medical Center, Box 359766, Seattle, WA 98104.
E-mail address: lsekhar@u.washington.edu (L.N. Sekhar).

Neurosurg Clin N Am 20 (2009) 453–485
doi:10.1016/j.nec.2009.07.007
1042-3680/09/$ – see front matter. Published by Elsevier Inc.

be possible.[4–8] With surgically inaccessible AVMs, embolization may be used to eliminate perinidal or flow-related aneurysms as a prelude to radiosurgery.[9,10] With large AVMs that are not candidates for surgical treatment, embolization may be performed in stages to reduce the size of an AVM and render it suitable for radiosurgery, in a protocol-driven fashion (the efficacy of this modality is as yet unproved). Several centers, however, have reported good preliminary experience.[9,11,12]

In general, any treatment of an AVM must offer patients a significant advantage over the natural history.[13] In this regard, the combined mortality and morbidity of procedures used must be considered in making a treatment decision and discussing options with patients.

The authors classify AVMs as ruptured and unruptured, because the natural history is different. The rebleeding rate of a ruptured AVM is 6% for the first year and 2% to 4% per year thereafter, whereas the bleed rate of an unruptured AVM has been estimated from 2% to 4% (as low as 2% and as high as 10%).[14,15] In addition, AVMs are generally classified according to Spetzler-Martin (S-M) grade (**Table 1**).[16] Although controversial, especially in regards to grade 3, which encompasses a variety of AVMs, it is the most widely used grading system. In this regard, the authors believe that the size of an AVM and its location (perirolandic, posterior fossa, or deep) are the most important variables determining outcome. The role of embolization-related complications has been well correlated with increasing AVM grade.[8,17,18] For S-M grades 1 and 2 AVMs,

embolization may be offered to mark an AVM for a surgeon (the black-colored Onyx [eV3, Irvine, California] is a good marker) to occlude an important feeding vessel that is surgically less accessible, to occlude a perinidal aneurysm, or to attempt to cure an AVM endovascularly. With grades 3 and 4 AVMs, embolization is usually performed in a staged fashion to reduce the risk of postoperative normal pressure perfusion breakthrough bleeding and to make surgery easier. Grade 5 AVMs are operated only under exceptional circumstances. For grades 4 and 5 AVMs, embolization may be performed as a prelude to radiosurgical treatment.[19]

With ruptured AVMs, the timing of embolization is a matter of variability and controversy.[8,20] In the authors' institution, patients with large clots are often operated emergently (if they are herniating and if an AVM is small) or early (within a few days). In such patients, embolization may be performed urgently if a surgeon desires. In other cases, embolization is started as soon as possible (without waiting for the clot to clear) and continued in stages (at approximately 2-week intervals) until the desired level of obliteration is needed.

Technique of Embolization—Brain Arteriovenous Malformations

Many centers have reported the safety and efficacy of N-butyl cyanoacrylate (NBCA) and particle embolization for AVM treatment.[21,22] Because of the well-documented handling characteristics of

Table 1 Spetzler-Martin grading score of AVM	
Characteristic	**Points**
Size of lesion	
Small (<3 cm)	1
Medium (3–6 cm)	2
Large (>6 cm)	3
Location	
Non eloquent	0
Eloquent site[a]	1
Pattern of venous drainage	
Superficial only	0
Any deep	1

Based on S-M grading system estimating the risk of surgery, which consists of three elements: size, venous drainage, and location. *From* Spetzler RF, Martin NA. A proposed grading system for arteriovenous malformations. J Neurosurg 1986; 65(4):476–83; with permission.

[a] Sensorimotor, language, or visual cortex; hypothalamus or thalamus; internal capsule; brain stem; cerebellar peduncles or cerebellar nuclei.

Onyx, however, the authors' institutional experience focuses primarily on Onyx embolization.

The majority of brain AVMs are now embolized with the liquid embolic agent, Onyx, in two viscous concentrations, Onyx-34 or Onyx-18. All embolization procedures are performed with patients under general anesthesia in a biplane angiographic unit. Systolic blood pressure during the procedure is controlled at less than 120 mm Hg. Post embolization, the blood pressure is kept 10% lower than the baseline systolic pressure in children or less than 110 to 120 mm Hg in adults after the procedure for 24 hours. After preparing and draping the groins in a sterile fashion, the femoral artery is accessed by an 18-gauge needle and, using the Seldinger technique, a 6-French (Fr) femoral sheath is inserted into the vessel and secured. Diagnostic angiography is then performed using a 4-Fr vertebral catheter with views of the intracranial (IC) vessels in various projections, including 3-D views, to delineate all feeders to an AVM and understand the dynamics of blood supply and venous drainage pattern. In some AVMs with rapid shunts, filming at high speed (6 frames/s) may be required. Intra- and perinidal aneurysms are noted.

Patients are heparinized before embolization, usually with 5000 U intravenously, and 1000 U per hour are repeated as needed to maintain the activated clotting time at 300 seconds (50 mg/kg in children). The heparin is not reversed at the end of the procedure unless there is intraoperative perforation of the vessel or rupture of AVM. The guiding catheter is constantly flushed via a pressure bag with saline, which does not contain any heparin.

The first vessel chosen for embolization is usually a direct feeder to the AVM (not feeding through collaterals and not an en passage vessel) with at least 2 cm of safe distance available for reflux before cortical branches are reached (**Figs. 1** and **2**A). A dimethyl sulfoxide (DMSO)-compatible microcatheter (Marathon 1.3-Fr eV3) is navigated into the artery close to the nidus of the AVM with aid of a 0.008-in micro–guide wire (Mirage, eV3); multiple reshapes of guide wire may be needed to reach the target site. In some cases, when an artery is large, a catheter may be able to be advanced along the vessel close to the AVM with the wire retracted inside, to avoid perforation of a thin-walled artery. It is important to have the microcatheter tip as close to the nidus as possible and to have a good distance between the catheter tip and any normal branch proximal to it (safe reflux distance). The safe reflux distance ideally should be at least 2 cm and clearly noted in the roadmaps before embolization. The micro–guide wire is removed and biplane superselective angiography is performed through microcatheter to analyze the anatomy of the nidus segment and verify that only the AVM nidus is filled. During embolization, good angiographic views of AVM in two projections should be shown on the screen to see the tip of the microcatheter clearly, to appreciate the reflux

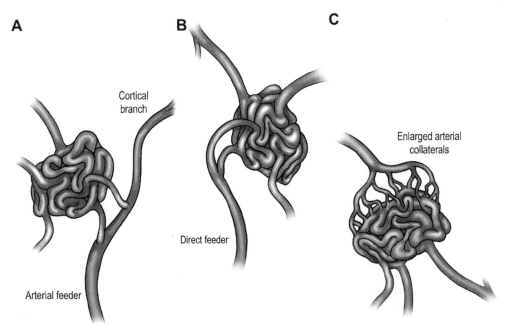

Fig. 1. Various types of feeder vessels to the AVM. (*A*) En passage vessel giving branches on its way to the cortex. (*B*) Direct feeder to the AVM nidus. (*C*) Network of enlarged collaterals supplying the AVM.

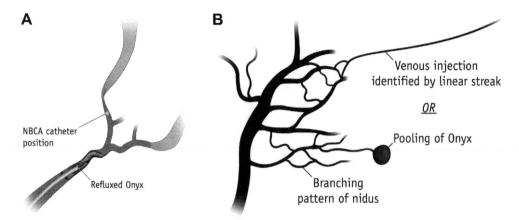

A

NBCA catheter
position

Refluxed Onyx

B

Venous injection
identified by linear streak

OR

Pooling of Onyx

Branching
pattern of nidus

Fig. 2. (*A*) Position of the microcatheter for Onyx embolization. Note the reflux of Onyx around the tip of the microcatheter to form a plug. (*B*) Patterns for identifying nidal injection and venous injection during Onyx injection.

readily, and to appreciate the anatomy of the AVM and the surrounding brain. Once embolization from this position is decided on, the microcatheter is over flushed with 10 mL of normal saline to clear any remaining contrast, then filled with 0.23 mL DMSO, and the catheter hub is also bathed in DMSO to clear the saline, because Onyx precipitates in contact with saline. Onyx is aspirated into a 1-mL syringe and a connection is made to quickly form a meniscus between the Onyx and DMSO. Onyx is injected slowly at a flow rate of 0.1 mL per minute to fill the microcatheter and replace the DMSO in the dead space. Embolization is usually started with Onyx-34 (twice as viscous as Onyx-18) in order to form a plug around the catheter tip. Free flow of the Onyx is noted into the AVM nidus until there is a reflux noted. Embolization is performed with a gentle and steady push, or gentle small puffs, with progress viewed all the time. In small AVMs, significant penetration may occur with the first push, before reflux occurs, so care should be exercised. When reflux is noted, the operator stops for varying periods of time (30 seconds to 1 minute) before restarting. After first reflux, anywhere from 2 to 10 minutes may be needed to form an adequate plug before the second forward penetration occurs again. As this point is about to be reached, forward and retrograde (bidirectional) flow often is observed.

Progress of embolization is followed by noting single radiographic exposures of the Onyx cast (and comparing with the AVM images) and intermittent angiographic runs to evaluate the AVM filling (**Figs. 3–10**). For each embolization sequence, a blank road map is obtained. Avoiding venous embolization is important. When passing through a vein, Onyx tends to laminate initially along the venous wall or quickly pass through to the venous sinus. During embolization, filling of the veins is noted by streaking or pooling, which is an indication to stop for up to 1 minute. The operator must have a good understanding of where the veins are inside the AVM and in its periphery to identify and avoid venous embolization. Reflux into normal brain areas around the AVM perimeter is an indication to stop for 30 seconds. The maximal safe reflux distance along the feeding vessel should be judged on the initial angiogram (usually no more than 2 cm back or 1 cm distal to a cortical branch of the feeding artery) and the fluoroscopy tube is appropriately positioned during embolization to judge this rapidly, because the embolic agent filling the AVM may interfere with the initial views. After the initial embolization epochs, with the plug well formed, the operator may switch to Onyx-18, which is less viscous and penetrates the AVM more easily.

Endpoint of embolization

Operators should use judgment and experience to end an embolization session. With small AVMs, the entire AVM or the majority of the AVM is embolized in one session. In such cases, the endpoint is reached when the major veins are filling (**Fig. 2B**). One should not try to achieve a perfect result with the sacrifice of safety, because this is when complications occur.

With large and giant AVMs, embolization is usually done in stages, with approximately 25% to 40% of the AVM embolized in the first session. The endpoint of an embolization session is reached when, after repeated pushes of embolic agent, no significant progress is noted. The considerations are to embolize larger AVMs (>3 cm) in a staged fashion to achieve maximal but safe reduction of the AVM volume and to embolize areas that are surgically difficult. The operator starts with direct feeders to the AVM (not en

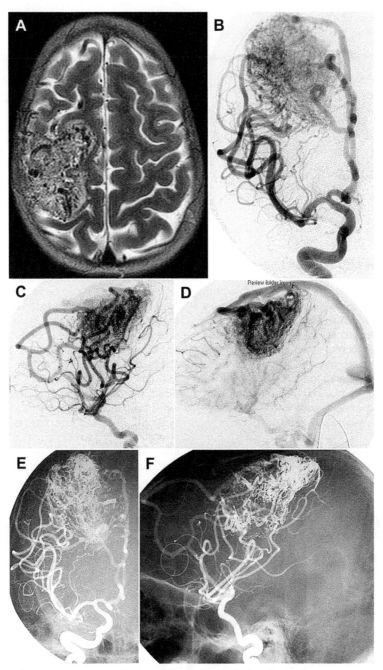

Fig. 3. (*A*) MRI scan showing a 7-cm AVM in the frontal lobe bordering the sensorimotor cortex. (*B*) Angiograms showing a S-M grade V AVM. (*C*, *D*) Angiograms showing Onyx cast obliterating the posterior portion of the AVM bordering the rolandic fissure after four stages of Onyx embolization in 3 weeks. (*E*, *F*) Plain skull radiographs show the embolized AVM.

passage feeders) and progresses to more surgically difficult areas. During subsequent sessions, the goal of an embolization should be to embolize regions that are more difficult for surgery (eg, the more posterior region in a perimotor AVM, the part supplied by the PCA branches in a parieto-occipital AVM, or the portion supplied by ACA feeders in a medial frontal AVM). With large AVMs, 2 to 3 days before surgical excision, a larger volume of the AVM may be embolized, but patients must remain in the hospital with strict control of the blood pressure until surgical resection.

Although it is preferable to embolize the apical portions of the AVM to make surgical excision

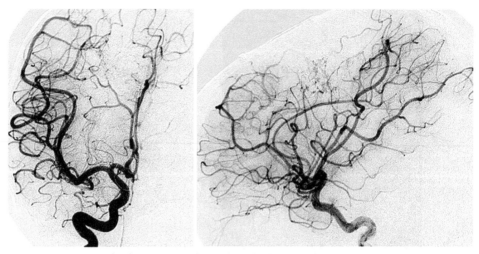

Fig. 4. Angiograms at 9 months showing complete removal of the AVM.

easier, this is often difficult, in the authors' experience. As much as possible, intra- and perinidal aneurysms must be obliterated in the first embolization session, especially in cases of ruptured AVMs. An embolization session is stopped when (1) the desired volume of embolization has been reached, (2) there is repeated opacification of draining veins, (3) the maximum safe distance for reflux is exceeded, or (4) despite a moderate injection pressure, there is no forward flow of Onyx.[21]

Management of vessel perforation

During initial navigation of the microcatheter, penetration of the artery may rarely occur by guide wire or catheter. It can be recognized by an unexplained position (relative to the arterial anatomy) of the wire or catheter or, in extreme cases, by changes in a patient's vital signs. It can be confirmed by a small-volume contrast injection through a microcatheter or by angiography through a guiding catheter. Once this is recognized, the catheter (or wire) must be left in place while the heparin is reversed with protamine. After reversal, while the microcatheter is withdrawn, a small (0.1 to 0.2 mL) volume of Onyx is injected into the artery to seal the perforation. Further embolization may be done through another vessel if the feeding artery is well sealed, the

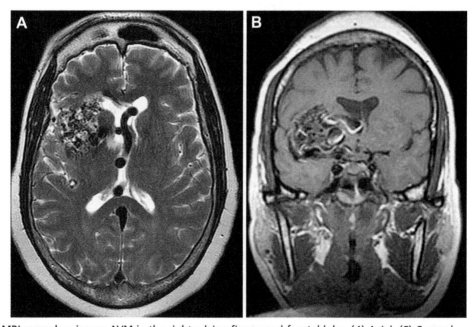

Fig. 5. MRI scans showing an AVM in the right sylvian fissure and frontal lobe. (A) Axial; (B) Coronal.

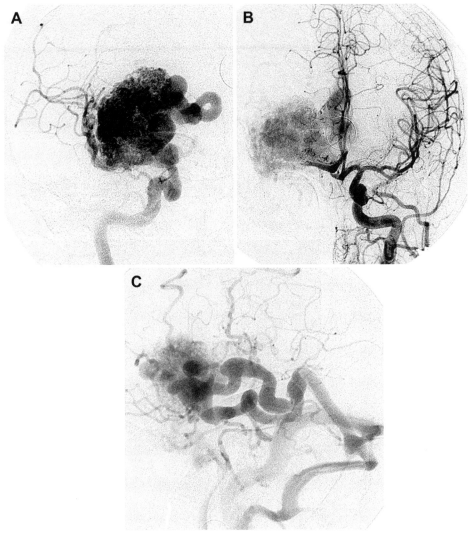

Fig. 6. Angiograms showing a S-M grade IV AVM with deep venous drainage. (*A*) Right carotid injection, antero-posterior view; (*B*) Left ICA injection, anteroposterior view; (*C*) Right ICA injections, lateral view showing venous drainage.

extravasation is minimal, and there are no changes in vital signs in a case of ruptured AVMs, or deferred to another session in cases of large extravasations, unstable vital signs, or unruptured AVMs. During embolization, extravasation of Onyx also may occur from the feeding artery, one of the draining veins, or inside the AVM nidus. This can be recognized by pooling and is an indication to stop the embolization.

Microcatheter withdrawal
At the end of the procedure, after aspirating with the Onyx syringe, the microcatheter is pulled back slowly, increasing the tension on the tip during withdrawal, holding the tension for a few seconds, and repeating this maneuver a few times until the microcatheter pulls out of the cast of Onyx

around it. During retrieval, protamine is kept ready for reversal of anticoagulation should an accidental rupture occur, but the authors have never had to use it in their series of patients. Immediately after retrieval of the microcatheter, the position of the guiding catheter must be checked because it can easily migrate cranially. The guiding catheter should be thoroughly aspirated to remove any clots before performing post procedural angiography.

Postoperative care of patients
Patients are monitored in an ICU, and the blood pressure is kept 10% lower than the baseline systolic pressure in children or less than 120 mm Hg in adults for 24 hours to minimize the risk of postembolization hemorrhage. Femoral sheaths

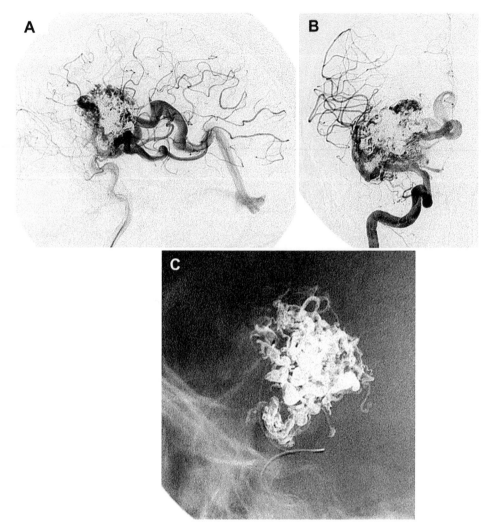

Fig. 7. Angiograms (*A*, *B*) and plain skull radiograph (*C*) showing the obliteration of the medial portion of the AVM by Onyx cast.

are usually removed on the following day and most patients are discharged home after 48 hours.

Hemorrhage from arteriovenous malformations during or after embolization and management

Hemorrhagic complications are devastating and probably occur due to inadvertent occlusion of the venous outflow during embolization without elimination of the arteriovenous shunt. Congestion of the nidus with slow-standing dye might be observed. Embolization of multiple pedicles at a single setting may result in too rapid an alteration of the hemodynamic of the AVM and may result in subsequent hemorrhage. This can be avoided by staged embolization. Finally, catheter/wire manipulation may cause vessel perforation resulting in intracerebral hemorrhage (ICH) or subarachnoid hemorrhage (SAH). This can be minimized by

limiting the use of guide wire to selecting the desired proximal pedicle while letting the natural flow characteristics of the AVM carry the pliable flow-directed microcatheter to the distal position for embolization. Immediate reversal of heparin with protamine and termination of procedure is required in arterial perforation with unstable parameters.

Arteriovenous fistulae

With very high-flow AVMs and arteriovenous fistulae, it may be necessary to use a larger Onyx-compatible microcatheter (Echelon 10 or Echelon 14, eV3) to allow the placement of coils into the vessel to arrest or slow the flow. This may be followed up with the liquid embolic agent. During such procedures, significant hypotension (down to 60-mm systolic blood pressure) or aden-osine-induced brief cardiac arrest may be used. In

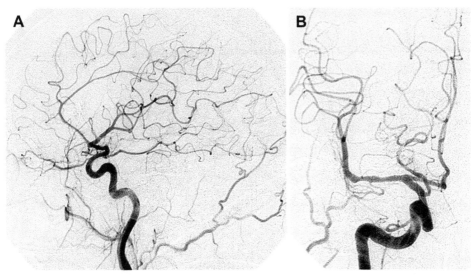

Fig. 8. Angiograms obtained at the time of follow-up showing complete obliteration of the AVM nidus. (*A*) Lateral view, right ICA injection; (*B*) Anteroposterior view, right ICA injection.

such cases, monitoring of somatosensory evoked potentials (SSEP) and motor evoked potentials (MEP) is helpful.

Clinical Experience and Outcome

In a series of patients treated by the authors' team from August 2005 to October 2008 at the their institution, a total of 128 patients were treated definitively, 4 by embolization alone, 60 by embolization and microsurgery, 14 by embolization and radiosurgery, 7 by all three modalities, and 43 by only surgical removal or radiosurgery.

From the total of 128 patients, 60 presented with rupture of the AVM and ICH or SAH. In a subset of 75 patients treated with embolization, complications were noted in 10 (**Table 2**). One patient developed left-sided hemiplegia 8 hours after embolization of a S-M grade V AVM in the occipitotemporal region through feeders from the anterior choroidal artery. She had an infarct in the right occipitoparietal and thalamic region on MRI. The AVM was surgically removed, but the patient remains disabled (modified Rankin score [mRS] 3). A second patient had an arterial perforation by the micro–guide wire that was managed by immediate reversal of heparin with protamine and termination of the procedure. She was successfully embolized the next day and had complete microsurgical resection after 2 more days. She had no neurologic deficits. Two patients had stuck microcatheters after embolizations that were left in situ; they were identified intraoperatively and extracted in both cases. There were two deaths of patients who did not recover after their bleed, unrelated to the treatment.

At 3 months, 63% recovered with no or mild disability. The outcome as measured by mRSs were slightly better in the radiosurgery series than in the microsurgery series in AVMS with S-M grades I to III but this difference was not significant ($P = .583$). One patient from the radiosurgery group had recurrent bleed in the interim period (**Table 3**).

Case Examples of Embolized Arteriovenous Malformations

Patient 1

An 8-year-old girl presented with recurrent tingling sensations on the left side of the body and weakness of the left arm and leg. She was found to have a S-M grade V AVM measuring 7.0 × 4.5 × 2.8 cm in size, involving the motor area. Embolization was aimed at the apex and the posterior part bordering the sensorimotor cortex parts of the AVM that were more difficult to manage with surgery. Onyx embolization was performed in four sessions over 3 weeks. The posterior portion of AVM bordering the rolandic fissure was embolized, but the apex could not be embolized. Surgical resection was elected because of her young age, which creates a greater potential for cerebral plasticity because she was likely to compensate for any deficits sustained at the time. The AVM was excised completely 4 days after the last stage of embolization. Postoperatively, she had increased weakness that gradually improved. At follow-up 3 years later, she had normal school and intellectual performance but a slight weakness of her left upper extremity with

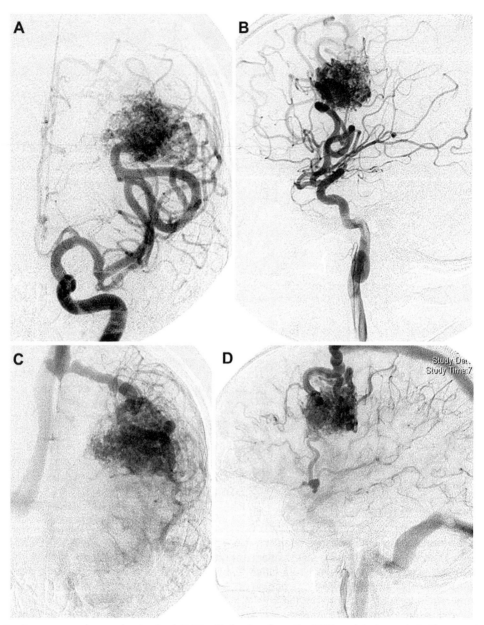

Fig. 9. Angiogram reveals a moderate-sized AVM with feeders from the MCA and drainage in to the superior sag-gital. (*A*) Left ICA injection, anteroposterior view, arterial phase; (*B*) Lateral view, arterial phase; (*C*) Anteropos-terior view, venous phase; (*D*) Lateral view, venous phase.

mRS 1, and angiography showed complete removal of the AVM.

Patient 2
A 52-year-old woman presented with recurrent severe headaches. She was found to have a S-M grade IV AVM in the right sylvian fissure, the basal ganglia, and the frontal lobe (see **Figs. 5** and **6**). Embolization was performed with Onyx in four sessions over 4 weeks, aiming at the medial portion of the AVM in the basal ganglia (see **Fig. 7**). Surgery was performed 2 days after the last embolization, and the AVM was removed completely. The patient had left hemiparesis post-operatively and had inpatient rehabilitation. At a follow-up examination 8 months after surgery, power in all four limbs was normal, and she had re-turned to her normal activities and work (mRS 1). Angiography 8 months after surgery showed complete obliteration.

Patient 3
A 22-year-old man presented with seizures. On imaging, he was found to have left frontal S-M

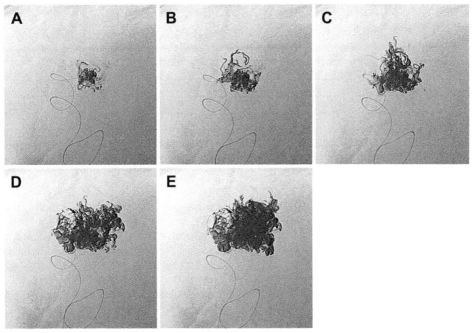

Fig. 10. Progression of the Onyx cast in various stages seen filling the AVM. Figures *A–E* are images of the ONYX cast during the embolization.

grade 3 AVM in the premotor area. He was subjected to two sessions of embolization with Onyx followed by surgical resection. Patient had a complete recovery with no symptoms at follow-up (mRS 0).

Patient 4

A 39-year-old man presented with intraventricular hemorrhage and on imaging was found to have thalamic AVM. The source of hemorrhage was a small perinidal aneurysm, which was then embolized to eliminate immediate rebleeding risk. He was subsequently referred for radiosurgery and patient is being followed up.

Patient 5

A 52-year-old man developed severe headache secondary to SAH with left cerebellar intraparenchymal hemorrhage due to AVM rupture. Angiography demonstrated a left cerebellar complex, racemose hemispheric arteriovenous malformation, predominantly fed by branches of the left posterior inferior cerebellar artery (PICA) with a perinidal aneurysm on the superior branch of the left PICA feeding into the AVM. Because of this, there was high risk of immediate rebleed and patient was planned for immediate embolization. He underwent preoperative embolization in two stages followed by surgical resection of the AVM and clipping of the superior cerebellar artery (SCA) aneurysm. Patient had a good recovery and was mRS 2 at follow-up.

DURAL ARTERIOVENOUS FISTULAS

IC DAVFs are acquired abnormal arteriovenous connections within the dura that account for 10% to 15% of all IC AVMs (**Figs. 11–23**).[23] Most lesions may develop as a consequence of venous sinus thrombosis and the attempted recanalization but some congenital DAVFs have also been described. There is a female preponderance with symptoms usually developing during middle to late adulthood. A presentation with aggressive neurologic symptoms is more common in men.[24,25]

Previous surgery, ear infection, and head trauma have all been cited as potential causes, although the common predisposing factor seems to be venous sinus thrombosis.[26,27] Venous thrombosis promotes venous hypertension, which acts as the initiating factor opening up microscopic vascular connections within the dura. Maturation of these channels secondary to progressive venous stenosis or occlusion results in the development of direct shunts between the arteries and dural veins.[28,29] In addition, a second complementary mechanism of DAVF evolution may occur with the release of angiogenic growth factors, such as vascular endothelial growth factor (VEGF) and basic fibroblast growth factor, promoting neovascularization and development of a DAVF.[30] Lasjaunias and Berenstein have suggested "an underlying dural weakness" facilitating dural shunts in some individuals.[31] In children, DAVFs may occur as congenital lesions, with

Table 2
Complications of embolization

Embolization	No. of Patients
Thromboembolic event leading to hemiplegia	1
Vessel perforation	1
Infection	1
Vein of Labbé stenosis	1
Stuck catheter	2
Failed catheterization	3

a presumed cause of venous thrombosis in fetal life or abnormal development.

Symptoms

DAVFs may be asymptomatic or present with symptoms that are mild to severe. Severe symptoms include ICH, visual loss, focal neurologic deficits, dementia, and eye pain or diplopia secondary to venous hypertension. Minor symptoms may include headache, tinnitus, dizziness, trigeminal neuralgia, hemifacial spasm, and so forth. Drainage of a petrous region DAVF to the transverse or sigmoid sinus commonly produces pulsatile tinnitus or hearing loss, sometimes in association with an audible bruit. Other cranial nerve (CN) symptoms (trigeminal neuralgia and hemifacial spasm) may be caused due to compression by an enlarged artery or draining vein. Cavernous sinus DAVFs may develop orbital signs, such as congestion, chemosis, and ophthalmoplegia.[32,33] More aggressive behavior may manifest as focal neurologic deficits, dizziness, a dementia-type syndrome or cerebral hemorrhage, including subarachnoid, subdural, or intraparenchymal bleeds. Such features are usually considered due to venous hypertension.

The most common location of cranial DAVF is transverse-sigmoid sinus followed by the cavernous sinus.[34–36] In a meta-analysis of 360 DAVFs, the tentorial incisura was the most ominous location, with 31 of 32 cases associated with hemorrhagic or nonhemorrhagic stroke.[32] The venous drainage pattern is the most important predictor of the clinical behavior, however, and those with retrograde leptomeningeal drainage

Table 3
Modified Rankin score outcome based on modality

Modified Rankin Score	Embolization/ Embolization + Surgery/surgery (%) N = 76	Embolization + Radiosurgery/ Radiosurgery (%) N = 52	Total No. of Patients (%) N = 128
0. No symptoms at all	25 (33)	14 (27)	39 (31)
1. No significant disability despite symptoms; able to carry out all usual duties and activities	24 (32)	20 (39)	44 (34)
2. Slight disability; unable to carry out all previous activities, but able to look after own affairs without assistance	12 (16)	7 (14)	19 (15)
3. Moderate disability walks without assistance	6 (8)	6 (12)	12 (9)
4. Moderately severe disability; unable to walk without assistance and unable to attend to own bodily needs without assistance	5 (7)	3 (6)	8 (6)
5. Severe disability requiring care	2 (3)	2 (4)	4 (3)
6. Dead	2 (3)	0 (0)	2 (2)

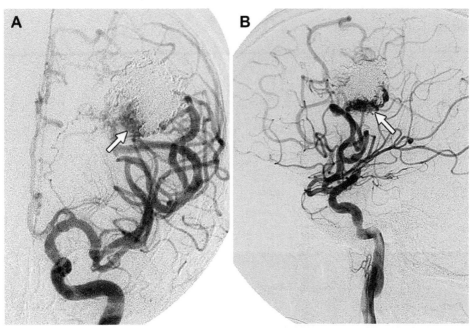

Fig. 11. After two stages of embolization, more than 70% obliteration of the AVM with only a small residual portion seen inferiorly (*arrows*). (*A*) Anteroposterior view, left ICA injection; (*B*) Lateral view, left ICA injection.

exhibit a much higher incidence of hemorrhage or venous infarction. The annual mortality rate for a DAVF with cortical venous reflux (CVR) may be as high as 10.4%, whereas the annual risks for hemorrhage or nonhemorrhagic neurologic deficits during follow-up are 8.1% and 6.9%, respectively, resulting in an annual event rate of 15%. Moreover, rebleeding rates may be as high as 35% over the first 2 weeks after the initial hemorrhage.[37,38] Thus, these formidable lesions need careful evaluation and rapid treatment.

The preliminary diagnosis of DAVF is based on clinical presentation. After initial suspicion, CT and CT angiography or magnetic resonance angiography may be performed. Angiography is needed for definitive diagnosis. The projections

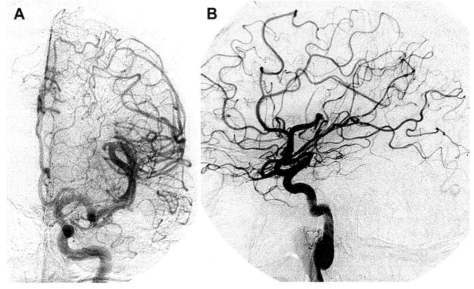

Fig. 12. Postoperative angiography shows complete resection of AVM with no residual AVM nidus seen. (*A*) Anteroposterior view; (*B*) Lateral view.

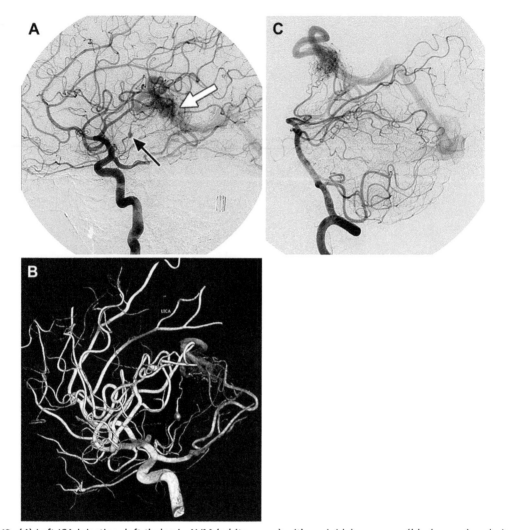

Fig. 13. (*A*) Left ICA injection; left thalamic AVM (*white arrow*) with perinidal aneurysm (*black arrow*) and nidus measuring approximately 2.4 cm × 1.4 cm × 1.7 cm centered in the left thalamus with left P1, P2, and P3 segment arterial feeders and drainage via the vein of Galen. (*B*) Three dimensional image of the left ICA injection showing the aneurysm; (*C*) Vertebral injection showing supply to AVM and drainage.

must include bilateral external carotid artery (ECA) runs, internal carotid arteries (ICAs), and both vertebral arteries (VAs) if necessary. For lesions around the foramen magnum, upper cervical area, thyrocervical, and ascending cervical arteries should be studied after an initial subclavian injection.

The Borden system of classification is commonly followed for classification and treatment indication, but the Cognard system is more detailed (**Tables 4** and **5**).

Treatment Philosophy and Algorithm

The primary goal of treatment is the complete obliteration of the lesion. In some cases, however, palliative treatment for control of symptoms may

be performed. The therapeutic armamentarium includes conservative monitoring, arterial embolization, transvenous occlusion, surgical excision, and radiation therapy. In current practice, many lesions can be eliminated by an endovascular technique. The main goal of endovascular treatment of aggressive DAVFs is to eliminate the cortical venous drainage and the resulting risk of ICH. Different endovascular approaches can be used in the treatment of these lesions.

In Borden 1 cases, treatment is needed only for severely symptomatic cases, and palliative (incomplete treatment) is an option. The aim of treatment in such lesions is cure, but palliation can be accepted to reduce the morbidity. In Borden 2 and 3 cases, treatment is mandatory, and when a patient presents after an acute ICH,

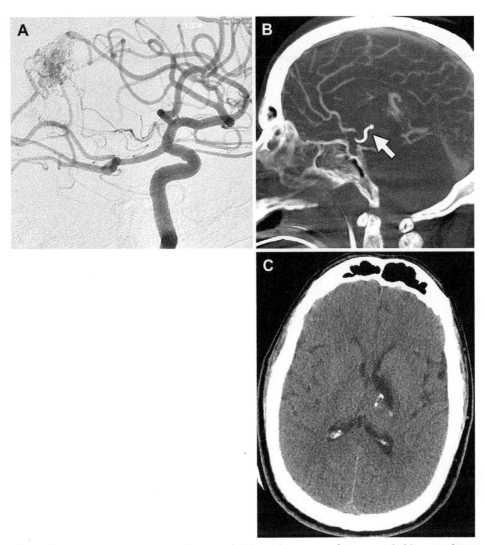

Fig. 14. (*A*) Carotid angiogram; reduction in the size of AVM and presence of Onyx cast (*white arrow*) post embolization. (*B*) CT angiogram; (*C*) CT scan without contrast.

treatment should be provided as soon as possible, to prevent the prospect of rebleeds. The goal is to occlude the fistula in all DAVFs, and especially to occlude the origin of the draining vein to prevent recurrence in Borden 3 fistulas. When endovascular treatment is difficult or has failed, then microsurgery is done as an alternative.[39,40] In some difficult cases, radiosurgery may follow the embolization procedure. In the authors' center, transarterial embolization with Onyx is used as the primary treatment modality unless there are arterial branches supplying CNs, predominant ICA feeders, or potential extracranial (EC)-IC collateral anastomosis. The transvenous technique is used in cases of type 2 DAVFs where transarterial access is not possible or where combined transarterial and transvenous treatment is needed. The goal of transvenous access is to enter the fistula

pouch from the venous side for coil embolization at the point of the fistula itself. In some cases of Borden 3 fistulas, the fistula can be accessed through the transvenous route.[41]

Surgical treatment is reserved in the authors' center for emergent clot evacuation and for cases where endovascular treatment is not possible or incomplete. A complete devascularization of the fistula or the occlusion of all the draining veins/vein of the fistula must be feasible for surgery to be successful.[41] Radiosurgery is performed as a last resort, for some cases of fistulae that cannot be optimally treated by one of the techniques described previously, usually after embolization or surgical resection. Radiosurgery takes 2 to 3 years to obliterate the DAVFs and, until the lesion is completely obliterated, there is still a risk of bleeding or other symptoms.[42,43]

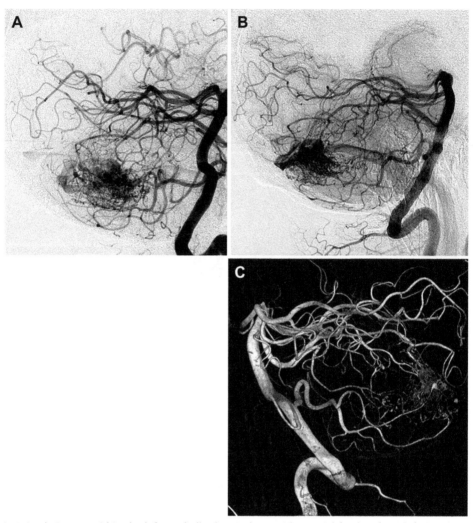

Fig. 15. S-M Grade 3 AVM within the left cerebellar hemisphere with arterial feeders from left AICA/PICA trunk, with small feeding branches from left superior cerebellar, and posterior cerebral arteries (*A, B*). Multiple small feeding artery perinidal aneurysms located close to the AVM nidus posteriorly (*C*).

Case Examples of Embolization Technique for Dural Arteriovenous Fistulas

Case 1: transvenous embolization of an indirect carotid-cavernous fistula

A 49-year-old man presented with headache and proptosis and was found to have an indirect carotid cavernous fistula (Borden 2) with bilateral meningohypophyseal trunk (MHT) feeders and left ECA feeders draining into the cavernous sinus, superior ophthalmic vein, and superior petrosal sinus. Complete obliteration of the fistula and relief of all symptoms was achieved after transvenous coil embolization of the cavernous sinus through the left superior petrosal sinus. This procedure was under general anesthesia, a 6-Fr sheath was placed in the femoral artery, and angiography was performed as needed during the procedure, using a 4-Fr vertebral catheter. The femoral vein was punctured, a 6-Fr sheath inserted, and a 6-Fr main pancreatic duct catheter negotiated into the internal jugular vein. An Excelsior SL-10 microcatheter (Boston Scientific, Natick, MA) with a Synchro 14 microwire (Target Therapeutics/Boston Scientific, Fremont, California) was then used to superselectively catheterize the left superior petrosal sinus and ultimately the left cavernous sinus. The catheter was positioned anteriorly at the junction of the left ophthalmic vein and multiple entering arterial fistula pedicles and multiple guglielmi base detachable (GDC) 360 platinum coils were deployed within the anterior left cavernous sinus. Occlusion of the fistula was confirmed by transarterial angiography.

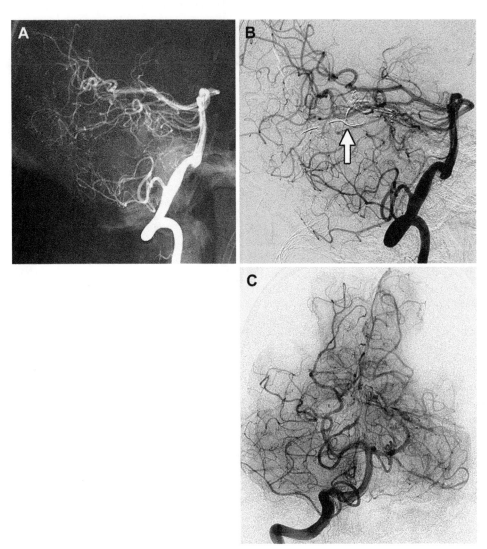

Fig. 16. (*A*) Postembolization showing significant reduction in the size of AVM. Postoperative angiography shows a complete resection with aneurysm clip seen in situ (*arrow*) (*B, C*).

The cavernous sinus is usually entered by navigating a microcatheter through the inferior or superior petrosal sinus. Rarely, when such access is not possible, and when there is predominant anterior drainage, catheterization can be via the superior ophthalmic vein or a facial vein. The superior ophthalmic vein can be exposed by a cutdown technique.

Case 2: transarterial Onyx embolization of convexity dural arteriovenous fistula (Borden 3)

A 60-year-old man presented with headache and was found to have an ICH. Cerebral angiogram showed a convexity osteo-DAVF with feeders from bilateral occipital artery, middle meningeal trunk, and right posterior cerebral artery. The venous drainage was predominantly into meningeal and cortical vein and into the middle third of superior sagittal sinus. There was partial narrowing of the superior saggital sinus and with venous congestion on bilateral ICA injections. Transfemoral access was achieved using a 6-Fr sheath under anesthesia. Superselective catheterization of the ECA was done using a 5-Fr Envoy catheter advanced over a 0.035 in glidewire. Using road mapping guidance, a Marathon 1.3-Fr microcatheter was advanced over a Mirage 0.008 microwire, and transarterial Onyx embolization was performed in three sessions through bilateral posterior branches of middle meningeal trunks and right occipital artery. There were no complications or CN palsies and the fistula was completely obliterated.

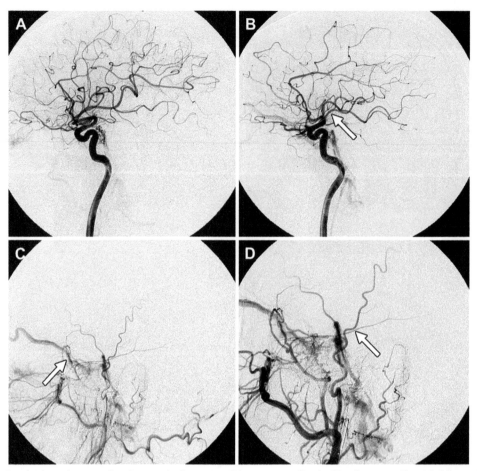

Fig. 17. Cerebral angiogram showing an indirect carotid-cavernous fistula (Borden type 2) with bilateral MHT feeders (*A, B*) and left ECA feeders (*C, D*) draining into the cavernous sinus, superior ophthalmic vein and superior petrosal sinus (*arrow*).

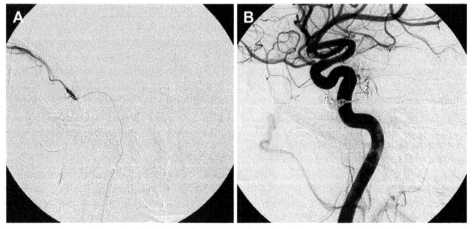

Fig. 18. (*A*) Tranvenous access to the fistula site through the left superior petrosal sinus. (*B*) Postembolization cerebral angiogram showing complete obliteration of the fistula.

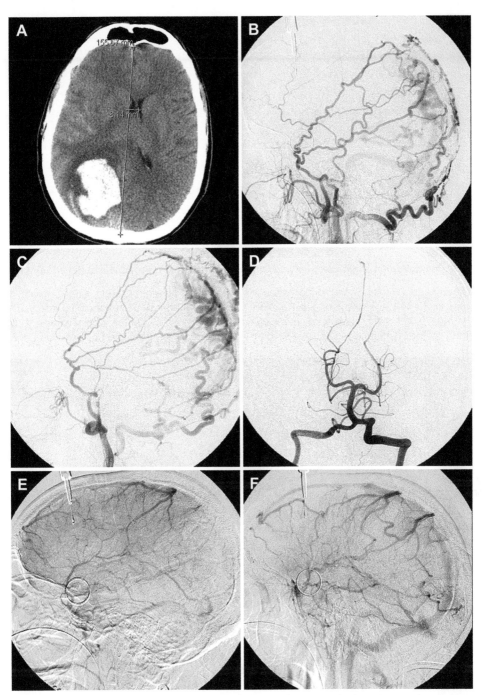

Fig. 19. (*A*) Noncontrast head CT showing an intracerebral hemorrhage. Cerebral angiogram showing a convexity osteo-DAVF with feeders from bilateral occipital artery, middle meningeal trunk (*B, C*) and right posterior cerebral artery (*D*). Venous phase of cerebral angiogram showing partial narrowing of the superior sagittal sinus and with venous congestion on bilateral ICA injections (*E, F*).

Case 3: Onyx embolization of tentorial arteriovenous fistula (Borden 3)

An 85-year-old woman presented with headache and was found to have a posterior fossa hemorrhage on CT scan. Cerebral angiogram showed

a tentorial DAVF supplied by feeders from bilateral occipital artery and left posterior meningeal branches. The venous drainage was into a tentorial vein that had a venous aneurysm and drained into the transverse sinus. A 6-Fr KSAW Shuttle-Select

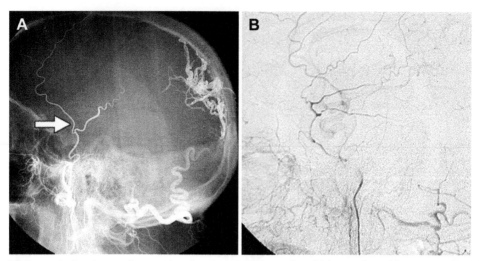

Fig. 20. (*A*) Postembolization angiogram showing Onyx cast (*arrow*) and (*B*) complete obliteration of the fistula.

(Cook, Bloomington, Indiana) introducer sheath was placed in the left ICA and using a Echelon 10 and Mirage 0.008 inch guide wire, compete obliteration of the fistula was achieved after

transarterial embolization with Onyx-18 through the dural branch of the occipital artery. The catheter was stuck in the occipital artery, broke at a point 10 cm from the tip, and was deposited in

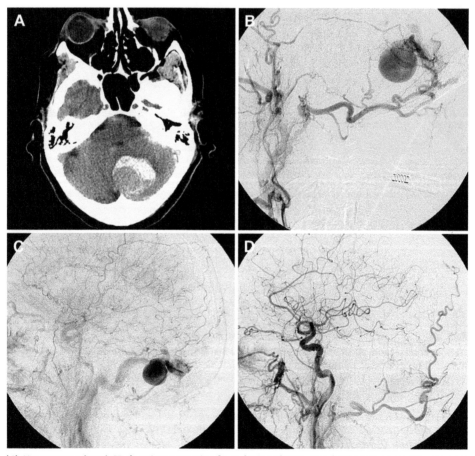

Fig. 21. (*A*) Noncontrast head CT showing posterior fossa hemorrhage. Cerebral angiogram showing a tentorial DAVF supplied by feeders from bilateral occipital artery (*B, D*) and left posterior meningeal branches. The venous drainage was into a tentorial vein that had a venous aneurysm and drained into the transverse sinus (*C*).

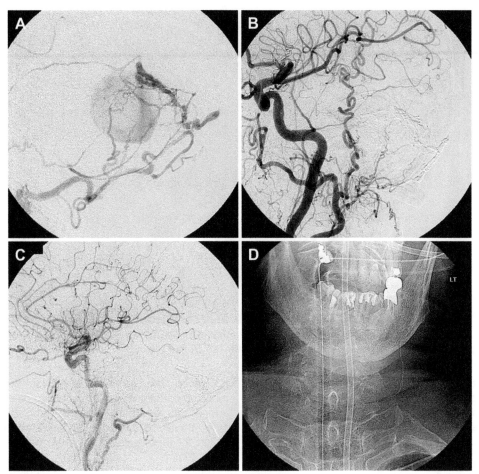

Fig. 22. Cerebral angiogram with selective left occipital artery injection (*A*). Postembolization angiogram showing complete obliteration of the fistula (*B, C*) and the retained stuck catheter (*D*).

the occipital artery after cutting the catheter just under the femoral skin edge.

Results and Complications

In the authors' institution, 32 patients with DAVF (**Table 6**) were treated over 3.5 years between May 2005 and December 2008 by endovascular embolization (transarterial embolization with Onyx, transvenous embolization GDC coils), surgery, or radiosurgery. Most common presentation was hemorrhage (n = 11), headaches, tinnitus, and orbital symptoms. Twenty-eight patients were treated by endovascular embolization. Five patients (after incomplete-1 patients/failed-4 patients embolization) had surgical excision of the fistula. Three patients were treated with gamma knife radiosurgery after partial obliteration of fistula with Onyx.

The distribution of patients according to Borden classification was I, 6 (18.8%) patients; II, 13 (40.6%) patients; and III, 13 (40.6%) patients.

Twenty-six of 32 (81%) patients had their fistulas completely obliterated after multimodality treatments at 1 to 36 months' follow up. Of the seven patients with residual after endovascular embolization, four patients had surgical obliteration of the fistula and three underwent gamma knife radiosurgery. Surgical complications included cognitive deficits with word-finding difficulty in one and seizures in another. At follow-up (3–36 months), 15 patients had mRS 0–2, four patients had mRS 3–5 (three due to the initial insult of the hemorrhage), and two patients were dead. One patient with a tentorial DAVF was attempted to be embolized by a transvenous technique, but the microwire was stuck to the vein during attempted extraction and caused its rupture resulting in massive hemorrhage and death. The other patient died after an accidental fall and consequent subdural hematoma (**Table 7**).

Transarterial embolization with Onyx has increased obliteration rates with low morbidity.

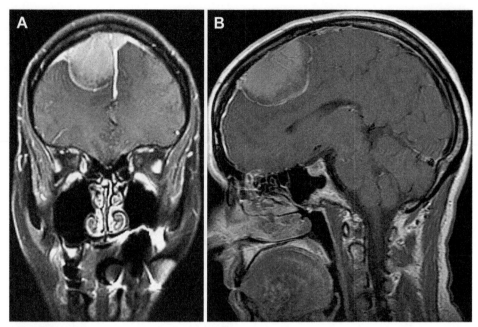

Fig. 23. (*A, B*) Postgadolinium T1-weighted coronal and saggital images showing a large right superior frontal meningioma with partial extension across midline into the left frontal region.

Surgical obliteration of the draining vein remains an important treatment option for fistulas not accessible through the endovascular route or after failed endovascular treatment.

EMBOLIZATION OF CRANIOCERVICAL TUMORS

Tumors of the craniocervical area are embolized mainly to make surgical resection easier, by reducing the bleeding during surgery, and sometimes, also by making them softer by inducing intratumoral necrosis (**Figs. 24–34**). Rarely, embolization can be used as a palliative modality to cause symptomatic improvement.[2,44–46] Because embolization is part of the multimodal treatment, it should be done with minimal risk, avoiding new CN deficits, stroke, or hemorrhage. Adequate devascularization of a tumor can rarely be produced without embolizing all the important feeders and the nidal portions of the tumor due to the presence of intratumoral collateral circulation. The vascularity of the tumor is often multicompartmental, as it is supplied by different arteries, but the intratumoral vessels do communicate with each other. At the conclusion of embolization, the feeding arteries may be occluded close to the tumor.[47]

Tumors that are considered for embolization are usually large and extra-axial, although embolization also may be performed of intra-axial tumors, such as hemangioblastoma, choroid plexus papilloma, or intraventricular meningioma, when the feeding arteries can be safely accessed. Extra-axial tumors considered for embolization can be divided into (1) convexity and parasagitta and (2) skull base tumors, the latter being technically more difficult.[34] In addition to intratumoral embolization, an endovascular surgeon may be asked to assess the risk of arterial sacrifice before or during surgery by the performance of a carotid occlusion test. Occlusion testing of a venous sinus is not safe and has been accompanied by a disastrous

Table 4	
The Borden classification system	
1	Venous drainage directly into dural venous sinus, no CVR
2	Venous drainage into dural venous sinus with CVR
3	Venous drainage directly into subarachnoid veins (CVR only)

Data from Borden JA, Wu JK, Shucart WA. A proposed classification for spinal and cranial dural arteriovenous fistulous malformations and implications for treatment. J Neurosurg 1995;82:166–79.

Table 5 The Cognard classification system	
Type I	Drainage into a dural sinus, with normal antegrade flow
Type II	Drainage into a dural sinus, with reflux into II a: (other) sinuses II b: cortical veins II a + b: sinuses + cortical veins
Type III	Drainage into cortical veins
Type IV	Drainage into cortical veins with cortical ectasia

Data from Cognard C, Gobin YP, Pierot L, et al. Cerebral dural arteriovenous fistulas: clinical and angiographic correlation with a revised classification of venous drainage. Radiology 1995;194:671–80.

complication in the senior author's experience (L.N. Sekhar, MD, unpublished data, 1992).

As with embolization of AVMs, endovascular surgeons and microsurgeons must communicate effectively to understand the goals of the embolization and the permissible risk before the procedure.

Embolization Technique

Diagnostic angiography

General endotracheal anesthesia is preferred for all embolization procedures, although in cooperative patients, and when a single vessel is embolized, local anesthesia with conscious sedation can be used. Using the Seldinger technique, a 4-Fr sheath is inserted into the femoral artery and secured. With the assistance of a microcatheter and micro–guide wire, the appropriate first- or second-order vessel is selected and catheterized with a 4-Fr vertebral catheter. Standard practice, for most large tumors, is to perform a diagnostic angiogram of both ICAs, both ECAs, and one dominant VA to document the status of the anterior and posterior communicating arteries. Based on a tumor's location, all potential sources of blood supply must be studied, and any dangerous anastomoses between ECA and ICA or VA branches must be ruled out. 3-D angiography may be used to better delineate the feeding vessel but, in some cases, superselective angiography of

the feeding vessel with a microcatheter may be required, although this is usually best performed once a decision to proceed with embolization is made. Venous assessment is important when a tumor is compromising the dural sinus or jugular vein.[48]

Carotid occlusion test

If an ICA is encased by a tumor, particularly if it is encased and narrowed, then an assessment of collaterals may be requested by the operating surgeon. Two levels of assessment may be performed. In the authors' center, a surgical sacrifice of the ICA is rarely done without a concurrent bypass procedure. In such a case, the authors perform only a carotid compression angiogram. Cerebral angiography with manual ipsilateral common carotid compression with contralateral ICA injection (anteroposterior view needed, focus on venous phase, filling, and emptying) demonstrates the potential cross flow through the anterior communicating artery. A delayed venous filling and emptying is the best evidence of poor collateralization. An Alcock's maneuver, which involves carotid compression during injection of the dominant VA (anteroposterior and lateral views show the entire skull for lateral view), can show the posterior communicating artery and potential collateral

Table 6 Location of dural arteriovenous fistula	
Location	No. of Patients
Transverse-sigmoid	10
Petrotentorial	8
Parasaggital/falcine	3
Anterior fossa	1
Middle fossa	2
Torcula	1
Carotico-cavernous fistula	7

Table 7
Complications of endovascular procedure

Endovascular Complications	No. of Patients
Stuck catheter	3
CN palsy (V/VII)	1
Rupture of vein with death	1

flow. A carotid occlusion test is performed with the patient awake. The ICA is occluded in the C1-C2 segment with a 7-mm × 7-mm HyperForm balloon catheter (Micro Therapeutics, Irvine, California) through a 6-Fr guiding catheter for 30 minutes after systemic heparinization, and patients are observed for any neurologic deficits.[49] The authors also use transcranial Doppler monitoring of the ipsilateral middle cerebral artery during the balloon test occlusion. A 30% drop in velocities with the balloon inflated indicates only borderline collateralization, and a 40% decrease indicates that the degree of collateral flow is probably inadequate to support cerebral perfusion. It is also helpful to have patients on aspirin (325 mg) for 1 day preoperatively.[50]

Embolization

Once a decision is made to proceed with embolization, patients are heparinized. For ECA embolization, a 4-Fr vertebral catheter is used as a guiding catheter. Usually, a Renegade 0.021 inch ID microcatheter (Boston Scientific) with a 0.014 inch or 0.016 inch hydrophilic micro–guide wire (for 350- to 500-µm *polyvinyl alcohol* [PVA] particles) or

a Marathon microcatheter with a Mirage 0.008 inch guide wire (for 45- to 150-µm PVA particles) is navigated into the vessel of interest, as distally as possible, and beyond any important potential collaterals. In case of the middle meningeal artery, the operator needs to get past the petrosal branch, which supplies the facial nerve. With any ECA embolization, all collaterals to the ophthalmic artery should be studied carefully and avoided, because sometimes the opthalmic artery has an aberrant origin from the MMA. With the microcatheter in place, superselective angiography is performed to study the microvasculature, intratumoral collaterals, and the ease of reflux. The microcatheter is flushed with saline before the embolic agent is introduced. For ICA or VA branch embolization, arterial road maps are needed; therefore, the 4-Fr sheath is exchanged for a 6-Fr sheath, and a 6-Fr guide catheter is used.

The most common embolic agent is PVA particles, mixed with contrast material. Particles, sizes 150 to 250 µm, are used for better penetration of tumor supply.[47,51] In the case of ascending pharyngeal or posterior auricular artery embolization, however, which may be giving rise to the

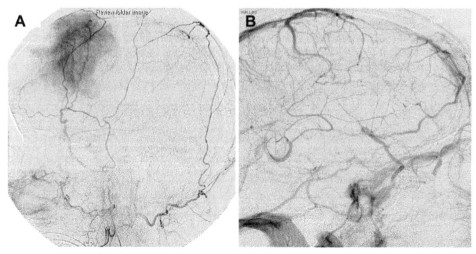

Fig. 24. An irregular area of moderate tumor blush is projected over the right frontal lobe supplied primarily from the frontal division of the right middle meningeal artery (*A*). A large area of filling defect is present within the adjacent superior sagittal sinus (*B*).

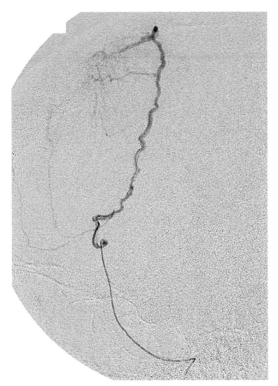

Fig. 25. Near complete stasis of flow within the frontal division of the middle meningeal artery with significant decrease in the previously noted tumor blush overlying the right frontal lobe.

neuromeningeal trunk supplying the CNs 9, 10, and 11, 350- to 500-μm particles are used. This avoids penetration of the fine blood vessels (vasa nervosum) supplying the nerves and attendant CN paralysis.[52,53] Embolization is performed in small puffs, with repeated road maps as necessary and continuous fluoroscopic observation, until stasis of contrast within the tumor is noted. At this point, the embolic syringe is replaced with saline, which is used to gently push out the contrast-particle mixture remaining inside the dead space of the microcatheter. In some cases of ECA embolization, the feeding vessel is occluded with Gelfoam torpedoes using Renegade microcatheter. Gelfoam supplied in sheets is cut into strips, approximately 1- to 2-mm wide and 2- to 3-mm long, and then rolled so that they are very thin. They are then loaded into the hub and the distal part of a 1-mL syringe, which is connected to the microcatheter, and injected.[2,47,51] They produce rapid occlusion of the feeding arteries, but recanalization occurs in approximately 6 weeks. The liquid embolic agent, Onyx, may also be used in cases of very vascular tumors; in such cases, the embolizaation technique is similar to that used for AVMs.

Embolization through the MHT is important in devascularizing clival meningiomas. When successful, and combined with embolization of any ECA feeders, this is effective in reducing the blood loss from these tumors.[54] The cannulation of the MHT may be technically demanding, often requiring 3-D angiography to understand the exact point of origin of the artery from the cavernous ICA and some probing with a microwire, with reshaping as needed. A Marathon 1.3-Fr microcatheter and a Mirage 0.008 microwire are used to cannulate the MHT, taking the microwire at least 5 mm past the origin of the MHT. Once cannulated with the microwire, difficulty may be encountered with the introduction of the microcatheter due to the size of the vessel or the angle of take off. When the microcatheter is well into the artery, it should be wedged at its branch point or slightly pulled back. Embolization is performed carefully, and with the smallest particles, to avoid reflux into the ICA and downstream embolization.

Embolization by Direct Puncture of the Tumor

This technique is rarely used when a tumor is difficult to access by the transarterial route but can be easily accessed by direct puncture.[55,56] Examples of this case are angiofibromas, paragangliomas, hemangiopericytomas, some tumors of the convexity, some jugular-mastoid tumors, and juvenile nasopharyngeal angiofibromas, particularly when the feeding arteries are not accessible due to previous procedures. The lesion is accessed through a prior craniotomy or a preauricular or precondylar area.[57] After selective transarterial angiography, the lesion is punctured and direct angiography is performed with and without manual compression of the venous drainage in the region and under fluoroscopic or ultrasound guidance. After the tumor is punctured, a contrast medium is injected through the needle to identify the corresponding tumoral compartment and its draining vein. Embolization is then performed with a mixture of NBCA (Cordis Neurovascular, Miami, Florida) and lipiodol (Guerbet France, Paris, France), injected using a 3-mL syringe under fluoroscopic control. NBCA and lipiodol are mixed in 1:3 proportions to which some powdered tungsten is added. With lipiodol, the progressive filling of the tumoral compartment can be followed visually with fluoroscopy. Several intratumoral injections are necessary to fill the tumor as completely as possible. Hence, the needle is withdrawn after each injection to reach another tumoral compartment. Each intratumoral injection must be slow and progressive, lasting from 20 to 30 seconds according to the size of the

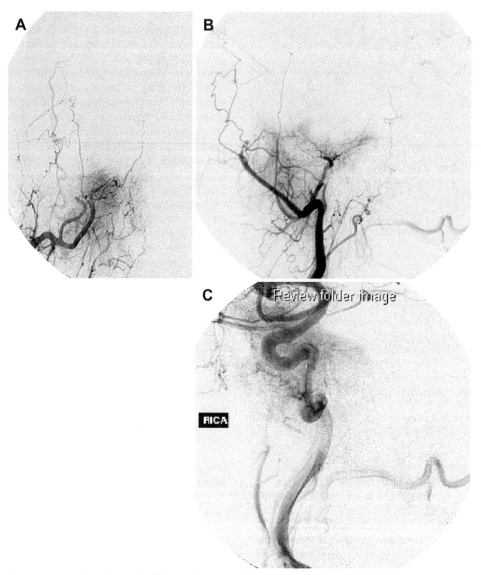

Fig. 26. Meningioma, primarily supplied by the right MHT (*C*), right middle meningeal artery, distal branch of the right internal maxillary artery (likely deep temporal) (*A*, *B*), and left MHT.

tumoral compartment. The injection is stopped when the NBCA starts to flow into the draining vein. In some cases, protection of ICA or VA is necessary with a balloon while using direct puncture embolization.

When Not to Embolize

The presence of dangerous EC-IC anastomoses, shared arterial supply between tumor and normal structures, the caliber of tumor vessel, and the potential for the embolic particles to reflux into the parent vessel are all factors that need to be considered before a decision to embolize.[52,53] Pial vessels are fragile and thus associated with

a high risk of arterial perforation and IC hemorrhage.[58] The potential for stroke due to thromboembolism when embolizing through pial vessels is also higher than when embolizing through ECA branches. If a major tumor blood supply is derived from small ICA branches or the ophthalmic artery, complete devascularization using microcatheters is not possible without unacceptable risk.

Complications of Intratumoral Embolization

Most common complications noted are fever and localized pain. Potentially more devastating complications include focal neurologic deficits due to inadvertent passage of embolic material

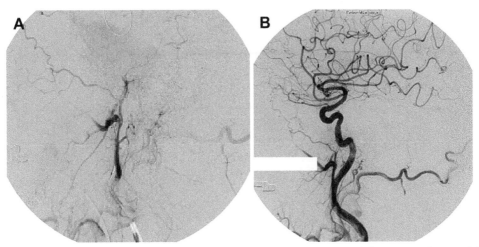

Fig. 27. Particle embolization of the right distal internal maxillary artery, right middle meningeal artery (*A*), right accessory meningeal artery, and right MHT feeding branch (*B*) with no residual significant tumor blush from the right ECA branches and very little residual tumor blush from the right ICA postembolization.

through reflux or from ECA branches through dangerous collateral anastomoses into the ICA or VA circulation,[47,50,52,53] and intratumoral hemorrhage. Embolization in the vascular territory of the ophthalmic artery carries a risk of blindness.[59] Cutaneous branches of the ECA may be occluded causing skin necrosis, thus complicating the prospective wound healing process.[59,60] Transient CN palsies (provided particulate reabsorbable embolic materials are used instead of polymerizing fluid materials) can also occur due to interruption of the vascular supply (vasa vasorum), which is often derived from ECA.[47,52] The petrous branch of MMA supplies the facial nerve and the neuromeningeal branch of the ascending pharyngeal artery supplies CNs 9 through 12 and can be inadvertently embolized. Tumor swelling post embolization may compromise the airway or increase the IC mass effect and this may be avoided by administration of steroids and early surgery after the procedure.[46,59–61] Shunting of the embolic material through the tumor in the setting of patent

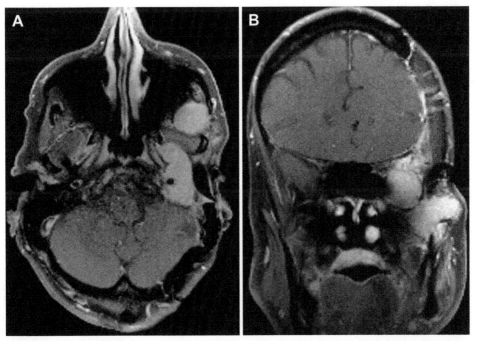

Fig. 28. MRI showing a hypervascular recurrent hemangiopericytoma in the middle cranial fossa. (*A*) Axial; (*B*) Coronal.

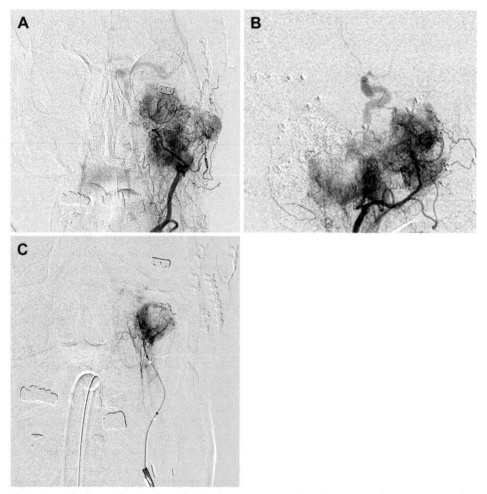

Fig. 29. There is marked vascular supply to lesion from two main branches arising from the internal maxillary artery and left occipital artery (*A*, *B*). Figure *C* is during the embolization procedure.

formane ovale may permit paradoxic embolization to occur systemically. A hypertensive response due to release of vasoactive peptides from large chemodectomas may occur and cause death. This can be avoided by careful anesthetic preparation and management.

Case Examples of Tumor Embolization

Patient 1: convexity meningioma with external carotid artery embolization

A 51-year-old woman presented with recent history of progressive headaches and memory problems. Neuroimaging demonstrated a large parafalcine meningioma, causing significant mass effect over the right frontal lobes. The tumor extended bilaterally across the superior sagittal sinus occluding it midway in its course. The patient underwent cerebral angiogram on the day before the operation and selective embolization of frontal division of the middle meningeal

artery supplying the tumor was done with 150 to 250 PVA particles through a 4F Renegade with a gold-tip microcatheter (Target Therapeutics/Boston Scientific) under careful negative road-map observation until stasis of flow was observed. She underwent a craniotomy and total resection of the tumor on the next day. Patient made a smooth recovery.

Patient 2: clival meningioma with meningohypohyseal trunk embolization

A 51-year-old woman presented with intractable seizure and on neuroimaging was found to have recurrence of petroclival meningioma. On angiography, there were feeders from bilateral MHT, right MMA, and distal IMA. Particle embolization was performed using a combination of 45- to 150-μm PVA particles in the right MHT and 150- to 250-μm PVA particles in the internal maxillary branches using a 6-Fr Marathon 1.3-Fr microcatheter . There was significant reduction in the tumor

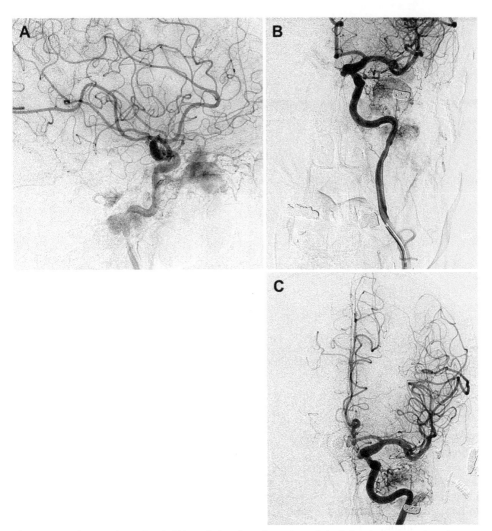

Fig. 30. There is vascular supply to the skull base lesion from branches of the inferolateral trunk and tumor vessels originating near the MHT. There is a prominent posterior communicating artery infundibulum. After embolization of the ILT and MHT vessels, the tumoral flush was significantly reduced (not shown)

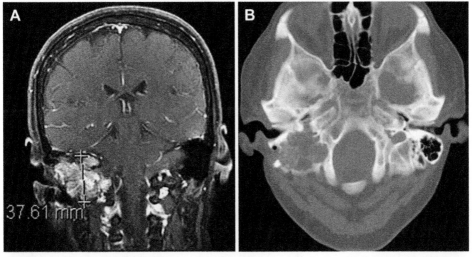

Fig. 31. (*A*) Coronal gadolinium MRI showing a contrast enhancing right mastoid mass lesion up to 4.1 cm in size. (*B*) CT with bone windows showing significant bone erosion.

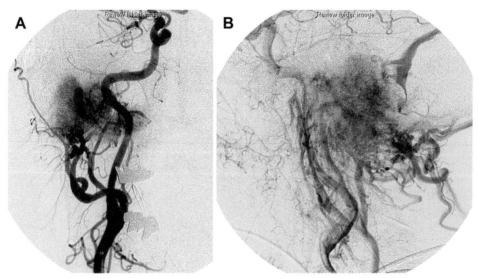

Fig. 32. Angiography revealed on right carotid injection a prominent tumor stain corresponding to the known right mastoid tumor. Early venous drainage is present and suggestive of arteriovenous shunt within the tumor. The tumor angiographic appearance suggests intraosseous meningioma.

blush after the procedure and she underwent surgical resection of the tumor.

Patient 3: recurrent hemangiopericytoma with embolization

A 58-year-old man with recurrent hemangiopericytoma who underwent multiple resections and gamma knife radiosurgery for his tumor was subjected to balloon occlusion test and embolization of tumor subsequently. In two sessions, embolization was done. The 6-Fr Envoy catheter was placed into the left ECA and an Excelsior 10 microcatheter (eV3) with the assistance of Synchro 14 microwire was advanced into an anterior and posterior division of the left internal maxillary artery and occipital artery supplying the tumor, and PVA particle embolization was carefully performed using 150- to 250-μm particles and negative roadmap technique. A large area of irregular tumor blush within the left aspect of the skull base

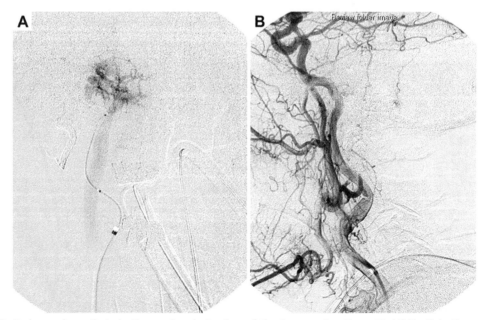

Fig. 33. Endovascular catheterization and embolization of the tumor using Onyx-18. (A) Postinjection angiography in the external carotid system demonstrated near-complete devascularization of the tumor (B).

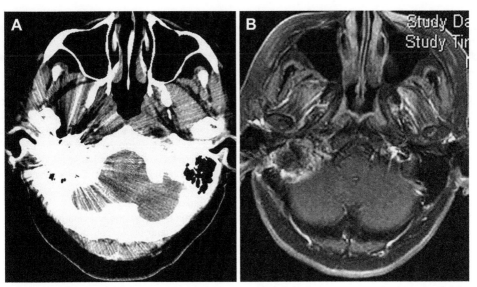

Fig. 34. (*A*) Postembolization CT scan shows presence of Onyx in the mastoid tumor and (*B*) post gadolinium axial MRI shows Onyx with central necrosis of the tumor.

supplied by branches of the ILT and vessels near the MHT from the left ICA and AICA were also embolized. After particle embolization of the said ECA and ICA branches, there was stasis of flow within these vessels and markedly decreased tumor blush.

Patient 4: tumor with Onyx embolization

A 62-year-old woman presented with history of headaches and was discovered to have a large hypervascular tumor. She had a previous surgery for Meniere's disease. Preoperative CT scan demonstrated significant bony erosion. MRI demonstrated multiple vascular flow voids. Angiography demonstrated the mastoid tumor as extremely vascular with prominent blush. Early venous drainage was suggestive of arteriovenous shunt within the tumor. The tumor was embolized using Onyx-18, PVA, and Gelfoam pledgets/torpedoes before surgery to reduce the extent of bleeding and reduce CN morbidity.

Results and Complications

At the authors' institution over the last 3.5 years, 18 convexity tumors, 42 skull base lesions, 19 intrinsic brain tumors, and 23 EC neoplasms were embolized by the endovascular team. Such embolization often, but not always, resulted in the reduction of bleeding during surgery and enhanced the ease of removal. There were no major complications encountered in the authors' experience.

SUMMARY

Endovascular procedures are rapidly expanding as treatment options for cerebrovascular diseases and neoplasms of the head and neck and are becoming less invasive but more effective. There are potentially dangerous anastomoses between the EC and IC circulations; hence, thorough knowledge of the anatomy is essential to minimize the risk of CN palsies, blindness, or neurologic deficits. It is essential to understand the scientific basis of treatment rationale based on advancing new neuroimaging techniques to better serve patients. An interdisciplinary approach and treatment in high volume centers are vital to obtain maximal benefit for patients.

REFERENCES

1. Dawbain RH. The starvation operation for malignancy in the external carotid area. JAMA 1904;17:792–5.
2. Macpherson P. The value of preoperative embolization of meningioma estimated subjectively and objectively. Neuroradiology 1991;33:334–7.
3. Manelfe C, Lasjaunias P, Ruscalleda J. Preoperative embolization of intracranial meningiomas. AJNR Am J Neuroradiol 1986;7:963–72.
4. Martin NA, Khanna R, Doberstein C, et al. Therapeutic embolization of arteriovenous malformations: the case for and against. Clin Neurosurg 2000;46:295–318.
5. Lundqvist C, Wikholm G, Svendsen P. Embolization of cerebral arteriovenous malformations: part II—aspects of complications and late outcome. Neurosurgery 1996;39:460–9.

6. Weber W, Kis B, Siekmann R, et al. Endovascular treatment of intracranial arteriovenous malformations with onyx: technical aspects. AJNR Am J Neuroradiol 2007;28:371–7.

7. Spetzler RF, Martin NA, Carter LP, et al. Surgical management of large AVM's by staged embolization and operative excision. J Neurosurg 1987;67:17–28.

8. Vinuela F, Dion JE, Duckwiler G, et al. Combined endovascular embolization and surgery in the management of cerebral arteriovenous malformations: experience with 101 cases. J Neurosurg 1991;75:856–64.

9. Gobin YP, Laurent A, Merienne L, et al. Treatment of brain arteriovenous malformations by embolization and radiosurgery. J Neurosurg 1996;85:19–28.

10. Henkes H, Nahser HC, Berg-Dammer E, et al. Endovascular therapy of brain AVMs prior to radiosurgery. Neurol Res 1998;20:479–92.

11. Dawson RC 3d, Tarr RW, Hecht ST, et al. Treatment of arteriovenous malformations of the brain with combined embolization and stereotactic radiosurgery: results after 1 and 2 years. AJNR 1990;11:857–64.

12. Dion JE, Mathis JM. Cranial arteriovenous malformations. The role of embolization and stereotactic surgery. Neurosurg Clin N Am 1994;5(3):459–74.

13. Ogilvy CS, Stieg PE, Awad I, et al. Special Writing Group of the Stroke Council, American Stroke Association. AHA scientific statement: recommendations for the management of intracranial arteriovenous malformations: a statement for healthcare professionals from a special writing group of the Stroke Council, American Stroke Association. Stroke 2001; 32:1458–71.

14. Ondra SL, Troupp H, George ED, et al. The natural history of symptomatic arteriovenous malformations of the brain: a 24-year follow-up assessment. J Neurosurg 1990;73:387–91.

15. Hernesniemi JA, Dashti R, Juvela S, et al. Natural history of brain arteriovenous malformations: a long-term follow-up Study of risk of hemorrhage in 238 patients. Neurosurgery 2008;63:823–31.

16. Spetzler RF, Martin NA. A proposed grading system for arteriovenous malformations. J Neurosurg 1986; 65(4):476–83.

17. Kim LJ, Albuquerque FC, Spetzler RF, et al. Postembolization neurological deficits in cerebral arteriovenous malformations: stratification by arteriovenous malformation grade. Neurosurgery 2006;59(1):53–9 [discussion: 53–9].

18. Hartmann A, Pile-Spellman J, Stapf C, et al. Risk of endovascular treatment of brain arteriovenous malformations. Stroke 2002;33(7):1816–20.

19. Steiner L, Lindquist C, Adler J. Clinical outcome of radiosurgery for cerebral arteriovenous malformations. J Neurosurg 1992;77:1–8.

20. Valavanis A, Christoforidis G. Endovascular management of cerebral arteriovenous malformations. Neurointerventionist 1999;1:34–40.

21. Natarajan SK, Ghodke B, Britz GW, et al. Multimodality treatment of brain arteriovenous malformations with microsurgery after embolization with onyx: single-center experience and technical nuances. Neurosurgery 2008;62:1213–26.

22. Velat GJ, Reavey-Cantwell JF, Sistrom C, et al. Comparison of N-butyl cyanoacrylate and onyx for the embolization of intracranial arteriovenous malformations: analysis of fluoroscopy and procedure times. Neurosurgery 2008;63(1 Suppl 1):ONS73–8 [discussion: ONS78–80].

23. Newton TH, Cronqvist S. Involvement of dural arteries in intracranial arteriovenous malformations. Radiology 1969;93:1071–8.

24. Sarma D, ter Brugge K. Management of intracranial dural arteriovenous shunts in adults. Eur J Radiol 2003;46:206–20.

25. Cognard C, Houdart E, Casasco AE, et al. Endovascular therapy and long term results for intracranial dural arteriovenous fistulae. In: Connors JJ, Wojak JC, editors. Interventional neuroradiology. 1st edition. Philadelphia: Saunders Company; 1999. p. 198–214.

26. Graeh D, Dolman C. Radiological and pathological aspects of dural arteriovenous fistulas. J Neurosurg 1986;64:962–7.

27. Watanabe A, Takahara Y, Ibuchi Y, et al. Two cases of dural arteriovenous malformation occurring after intracranial surgery. Neuroradiology 1984;26: 375–80.

28. Chaudhary M, Sachdev V, Cho S. Dural arteriovenous malformations of the major venous sinuses: an acquired lesion. AJNR Am J Neuroradiol 1982; 3:13–9.

29. Kwon BJ, Han MH, Kang HS, et al. MR imaging features of intracranial dural arteriovenous fistulas: relations with venous drainage patterns. AJNR Am J Neuroradiol 2000;26:2500–7.

30. Uranishi R, Nakase H, Sakaki T. Expression of angiogenetic growth factors in dural arteriovenous fistula. J Neurosurg 1999;91:781–6.

31. Lasjaunias P, Berenstein A, ter Brugge KG. Surgical Neuroangiography. 2nd edition. Springer; 2001.

32. Awad IA, Little RJ, Akrawi WP, Ahl J. Intracranial dural arteriovenous malformations: factors predisposing to an aggressive neurological course. J Neurosurg 1990;72:839–50.

33. Lasjaunias P, Chiu M, terBrugge KT. Neurological manifestations of intracranial dural sinus arteriovenous malformations. J Neurosurg 1986;64:724–30.

34. Cognard C, Gobin YP, Pierot L, et al. Cerebral dural arteriovenous fistulas: clinical and angiographic correlation with a revised classification of venous drainage. Radiology 1995;194:671–80.

35. Brown RD Jr, Wiebers DO, Nichols DA. Intracranial dural arteriovenous fistulae: angiographic predictors of intracranial hemorrhage and clinical outcome in nonsurgical patients. J Neurosurg 1994;81:531–8.

36. Halbach VV, Higashida RT, Hieshima GB, et al. Dural fistulas involving the cavernous sinus: results of treatment in 30 patients. Radiology 1987;163:437–42.

37. van Dijk JM, terBrugge KG, Willinsky RA, et al. Clinical course of cranial dural arteriovenous fistulas with long-term persistent cortical venous reflux. Stroke 2002;33:1233–6.

38. Duffau H, Lopes M, Janosevic V, et al. Early rebleeding from intracranial dural arteriovenous fistulas: report of 20 cases and review of the literature. J Neurosurg 1999;90:78–84.

39. Ushikoshi S, Houkin K, Kuroda S, et al. Surgical treatment of intracranial dural arteriovenous fistulas. Surg Neurol 2002;57:253–61.

40. Collice M, D'Aliberti G, Arena O, et al. Surgical treatment of intracranial dural arteriovenous fistulae: role of venous drainage. Neurosurgery 2000;47:56–66 [discussion: 66–7].

41. Caragine LP Jr, Halbach VV, Dowd CF, et al. Intraorbital arteriovenous fistulae of the ophthalmic veins treated by transvenous endovascular occlusion: technical case report. Neurosurgery 2006;58(Suppl 1):ONS-E170 [discussion: ONS-E170].

42. Koebbe CJ, Singhal D, Sheehan J, et al. Radiosurgery for dural arteriovenous fistulas. Surg Neurol 2005;64:392–9.

43. Soderman M, Edner G, Ericson K, et al. Gamma knife surgery for dural arteriovenous shunts: 25 years of experience. J Neurosurg 2006;104:867–75.

44. American Society of Interventional and Therapeutic Neuroradiology. Head, neck, and brain tumor embolization. AJNR Am J Neuroradiol 2001;22:S14–5.

45. Hekster RE, Matricali B, Luyendijk W. Presurgical transfemoral catheter embolization to reduce operative blood loss. Technical note. J Neurosurg 1974;41:396–8.

46. Chun JY, McDermott MW, Lamborn KR, et al. Delayed surgical resection reduces intraoperative blood loss for embolized meningiomas. Neurosurgery 2002;50:1231–7.

47. Ahuja A, Gibbons KJ. Endovascular therapy of central nervous system tumors. Neurosurg Clin N Am 1994;5:541–54.

48. Sekhar LN, Pomeranz S, Janecka IP, et al. Temporal bone neoplasms: a report on 20 surgically treated cases. J Neurosurg 1992;76:578–87.

49. Accreditation Council on Graduate Medical Education. Carotid artery balloon test occlusion. AJNR Am J Neuroradiol 2001;22(Suppl):S8–9.

50. Berdick TR, Hoffer EK, Kooy T, et al. Which arteries are expendable? The practice and pitfalls of embolization throughout the body. Semin Intervent Radiol 2008;25:191–203.

51. Qureshi AI. Endovascular treatment of cerebrovascular diseases and intracranial neoplasms. Lancet 2004;363:804–13.

52. Lapresle J, Lasjaunias P. Cranial nerve ischaemic arterial syndromes. A review. Brain 1986;109(Pt 1):207–16.

53. Lasjaunias P, Doyon D. The ascending pharyngeal artery and the blood supply of the lower cranial nerves. J Neuroradiol 1978;5(4):287–301.

54. Robinson DH, Song JK, Eskridge JM. Embolization of meningohypophyseal and inferolateral branches of the cavernous internal carotid artery. AJNR Am J Neuroradiol 1999;20:1061–7.

55. George B, Casasco A, Deffrennes D, et al. Intratumoral embolization of intracranial and extracranial tumors: technical note. Neurosurgery 1994;35:771–3 [discussion: 773–4].

56. Casasco A, Herbreteau D, Houdart E, et al. Devascularization of craniofacial tumors by percutaneous tumor puncture. AJNR Am J Neuroradiol 1994;15:1233–9.

57. Chaloupka JC, Mangla S, Huddle DC, et al. Evolving experience with direct puncture therapeutic embolization for adjunctive and palliative management of head and neck hypervascular neoplasms. Laryngoscope 1999;109(11):1864–72.

58. Kallmes DF, Evans AJ, Kaptain GJ, et al. Hemorrhagic complications in embolization of a meningioma: case report and review of the literature. Neuroradiology 1997;39:877–80.

59. Gruber A, Killer M, Mazal P, et al. Preoperative embolization of intracranial meningiomas: a 17-year single center experience. Minim Invasive Neurosurg 2000;43:18–29.

60. Adler JR, Upton J, Wallman J, et al. Management and prevention of necrosis of the scalp after embolization and surgery for meningioma. Surg Neurol 1986;25:357–60.

61. Halbach VV, Hieshima GB, Higashida RT, et al. Endovascular therapy of head and neck tumors. In: Viñuela F, Halbach VV, Dion JE, editors. Interventional neuroradiology: endovascular therapy of the central nervous system. New York: Raven Press; 1992. p. 17–28.

Endovascular Management of Extracranial Carotid and Vertebral Disease

Hjalti M. Thorisson, MD[a,b], Michele H. Johnson, MD[a,c,d,e],*

KEYWORDS

- Carotid stenosis • Epistaxis • Carotid blowout
- Carotid dissection • Endovascular management

The role of endovascular management in the treatment of extracranial carotid and vertebral vascular pathology is extensive and expanding. It is imperative for the neuroendovascular specialist to be proficient with diagnosis and treatment of common extracranial pathologies. For this discussion, we divide extracranial vascular disease processes into atherosclerotic and nonatherosclerotic vascular disease. The atherosclerotic disease discussion includes a review of clinical trials for symptomatic and asymptomatic carotid stenosis and surgical, medical, and endovascular treatments currently available. The nonatherosclerotic injury category encompasses trauma, vascular injury attributable to cancer or cancer treatment, spontaneous dissection and sequelae, and idiopathic epistaxis. Although these underlying pathologies differ, the diagnostic algorithm and therapeutic approaches are similar from the perspective of the neuroendovascular specialist.

ATHEROSCLEROTIC DISEASE
Extracranial Carotid Stenosis

Ischemic stroke is a major cause of morbidity and mortality in the western world. An estimated 8% to 29% of ischemic strokes are caused by extracranial atherosclerotic diseases (most frequently carotid bifurcation stenosis).[1] Current treatment modalities for extracranial cervical carotid atherosclerotic disease include medical management, carotid endarterectomy (CEA), and carotid angioplasty and stenting (CAS).

Carotid endarterectomy

Few surgical procedures have undergone the same rigorous scrutiny as CEA. Ever since its inception in the 1950s, CEA for the treatment of carotid bifurcation stenosis has generated debate with respect to appropriate use. In the 1980s, CEA was the most common vascular surgical procedure and questions regarding appropriate use led to large randomized trials both in North America and Europe to evaluate its efficacy for treatment of symptomatic and asymptomatic lesions. Carotid stenosis is considered symptomatic if there is a history of ipsilateral stroke, ipsilateral transient ischemic attack, or ipsilateral transient monocular blindness within the preceding 6 months.

Symptomatic carotid stenosis

The North American Symptomatic Carotid Endarterectomy Trial (NASCET) randomized

a Department of Diagnostic Radiology, Yale University School of Medicine, 333 Cedar Street, PO Box 208042, New Haven, CT 06520, USA
b Department of Radiology, University Hospital - Landspitali Haskolasjukrahus i Fossvogi, Reykjavik, Iceland
c Department of Surgery (Otolaryngology), Yale University School of Medicine, 333 Cedar Street, PO Box 208042, New Haven, CT 06520, USA
d Department of Neurosurgery, Yale University School of Medicine, 333 Cedar Street, PO Box 208042, New Haven, CT 06520, USA
e Interventional Neuroradiology, Yale University School of Medicine, 333 Cedar Street, PO Box 208042, New Haven, CT 06520, USA
* Corresponding author. Department of Diagnostic Radiology, Yale University School of Medicine, 333 Cedar Street, PO Box 208042, New Haven, CT 06520.
E-mail address: michele.h.johnson@yale.edu (M.H. Johnson).

Neurosurg Clin N Am 20 (2009) 487–506
doi:10.1016/j.nec.2009.07.011
1042-3680/09/$ – see front matter © 2009 Published by Elsevier Inc.

symptomatic patients from 50 centers to CEA with medical management versus medical management alone. Initial results were reported in 1991 and demonstrated a significant benefit to patients with high-grade carotid stenosis (70% to 99%) who underwent CEA.[2] The risk of an ipsilateral stroke over a 2-year period was 26% in the medical group but 9% in the CEA group, representing an absolute risk reduction for the surgical arm of the study of 17% decreased risk of any ipsilateral stroke over a 2-year period. These results were essentially corroborated in the European Carotid Surgery Trial (ECST) in 1998.[3] Accounting for differences in angiographic quantitation of carotid stenosis, the results of NASCET and ECST were in agreement that CEA was of clear benefit to symptomatic patients with carotid stenosis between 70% and 99% (when measured using the NASCET criteria).[4] Further results of the NASCET study published in 1998 showed that symptomatic patients with moderate stenosis (50% to 69% by NASCET criteria) also benefit from CEA,[5] although that benefit was less striking and more apparent in men than women. These studies established the legitimacy of CEA for treatment of symptomatic carotid stenosis greater than 70%.

Asymptomatic carotid stenosis

The NASCET and ECST studies did not address the increasingly large, asymptomatic population diagnosed with carotid stenosis by imaging. The Asymptomatic Carotid Atherosclerosis Study group (ACAS) trial, published in 1995, randomized 1662 patients with greater than 60% carotid stenosis to CEA with medical management versus medical management alone and found an estimated absolute risk reduction in the surgically treated group of 5.9% in the risk of ipsilateral stroke over a 5-year period as compared with medical management alone. These results were further corroborated by the Asymptomatic Carotid Surgery Trial (ACST) published in 2004 that also showed a 6% absolute risk reduction of ipsilateral stroke over a 5-year period in the surgically treated group. Bear in mind that the patients randomized in the ACAS trial were highly selected, with multiple exclusion criteria (age older than 80, significant medical morbidities, and more), and in addition, the surgeons performing the CEA had to show a perioperative complication rate of less than 3% to be allowed to participate in the study.[6,7] Previous trials had failed to show a benefit for CEA in asymptomatic patients (Veterans Affairs trial[8] and the Mayo Clinic trial[9]). The American Heart Association guidelines for treatment recommend CEA for symptomatic extracranial carotid stenosis (>70%) if the periprocedural rate of major stroke or death was under 6% and treating asymptomatic extracranial carotid stenosis (>70%) if the periprocedural rate of major stroke and death was under 3% and the life expectancy of the patient was at least 5 years.[10] Also of significance, best medical management has improved significantly since these trials were performed, with a more defined role for statin therapy, angiotensin-converting enzyme (ACE) inhibitors, and added antiplatelet therapy.

Carotid angioplasty and stenting

Initial endovascular treatment of extracranial carotid artery stenosis involved percutaneus balloon angioplasty with isolated case reports and small series published in the early 1980s.[11] The touted benefits of endovascular treatment included minimally invasive approach allowing treatment of patients with severe cardiac and pulmonary disease, decreased cranial nerve injury, and suitablility for patients with anatomically difficult lesions for a surgical approach and in patients with a prior history of neck radiation. Although CAS does avoid some of the complications associated with CEA, such as cranial nerve injury, there are specific procedural risks that are unique, such as groin or retroperitoneal hematoma, vessel dissection related to catheterization and contrast reaction, as well as the risk of stroke. There are anatomic configurations unfavorable for CAS such as severe tortuosity of the carotid vessels, or severe angulation between the aortic arch and origin of the brachiocephalic or carotid arteries (**Fig. 1**). It very quickly became apparent that the major limitation of endovascular treatment was the risk of embolic stroke that initially seemed significantly higher for patients treated with percutaneous transluminal angioplasty (PTA) with or without stenting versus those treated with surgery.[12]

Randomized controlled trials of carotid endarterectomy versus carotid angioplasty and stenting

When evaluating the literature comparing CEA and CAS, several issues must be considered:

1. Case series registries versus randomized controlled trials (RCTs)
2. Symptomatic versus asymptomatic patients
3. Low-risk surgical candidates versus high-risk surgical candidates (and thus would have been excluded from the relevant surgical trials)
4. Periprocedural medical management
5. Use of cerebral protection device during CAS
6. Operator experience

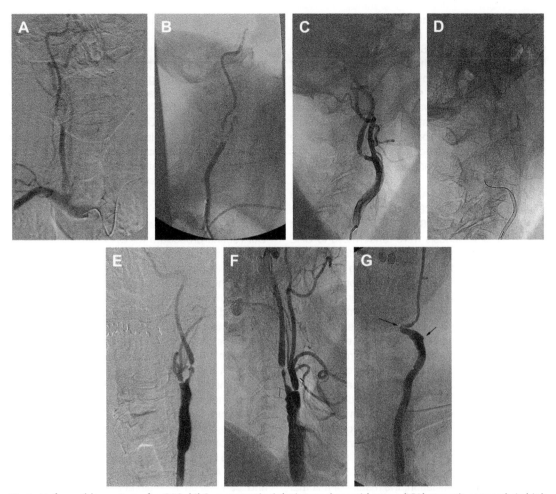

Fig. 1. Unfavorable anatomy for CAS. (*A*) Symptomatic right internal carotid artery (ICA) stenosis accessed via high left brachial approach owing to occlusive vascular disease in the femoral arteries. (*B*) Although diagnostic angiography was successful, the shuttle sheath could not be advanced into a position suitable for stent placement. (*C*) Symptomatic right ICA stenosis with tortuosity of the common carotid artery. (*D*) The tortuosity at the arch and the angle of the right ICA origin prevented advancement of the protection device beyond the origin of the guiding catheter. The procedure was aborted and an awake endarterectomy performed. (*E, F*) Distal patch graft stenosis involves both internal and external carotid arteries, however there is a marked disparity in size between the graft and the internal carotid artery precluding stent placement. (*G*) The external carotid artery is occluded in this patient with oral bleeding and recurrent tonsilar cancer. The size disparity between the common and internal carotid arteries and the acuteness of the angled precluded stent placement and the vessel was permanently occluded with coils.

The first RCT comparing CEA and CAS was published in 1998 and was a small trial that was stopped prematurely because of a very high incidence (70%) of stroke in the CAS arm of the trial.[12] The Carotid And Vertebral Transluminal Angioplasty Study (CAVATAS) was published in 2001 and showed no significant difference in 30-day morbidity and mortality rates when comparing CEA and CAS.[13] However, complication rates in both groups were high by conventional standards, with a 30-day death or disabling stroke rate of 10.0% and 9.9% for CAS and CEA respectively. Only about a quarter of endovascularly treated

patients received a stent and restenosis rates were higher in the endovascular group.

The first RCT in high-risk patients was the Stenting and Angioplasty with Protection in Patients at High Risk for Endarterectomy (SAPPHIRE) trial published in 2004.[14] Patients randomized for the trial would likely have been excluded from the large surgical trials because of age and/or comorbidity. Only experienced surgeons and interventionalists were allowed to participate in the trial. Most of the patients were asymptomatic (about 70% in both arms); embolic protection devices and stents were used in the endovascular arm of the study. The results showed a significantly lower 30-day mortality/major stroke/myocardial infarction (MI) rate in the CAS group (4.8%) versus the CEA group (9.8%) and this benefit was still present at 1 year after intervention. However, it is important to realize that the vast majority of the difference between the two arms was because of a difference in the rate of MI (most MIs were non–Q-wave infarctions detected on routine postoperative tests). If MI is excluded as an end point, there was no statistically significant difference between groups.

The Stent Protected Angioplasty versus Carotid Endarterectomy (SPACE) trial was published in 2006.[15] A total of 1183 symptomatic patients with over 70% stenosis were randomized to CAS or CEA. Use of embolic protection devices was left to the discretion of the treating physician. Results showed a similar rate of complications between the groups. The 30-day mortality/major stroke rate was 6.8% in the CAS arm and 6.3% in the CEA arm. The authors concluded that CEA was still the gold standard because evidence of the equivalence or superiority of endovascular treatment is lacking. The Endarterectomy Versus Stenting in Patients with Symptomatic Severe Carotid Stenosis (EVA-3S) was also published in 2006. After randomizing 527 patients to CAS or CEA, the trial was stopped because of concerns regarding the safety of CAS. Periprocedural 30-day mortality and major stroke rates were 9.6% in the CAS arm compared with 3.9% in the CEA arm. Since publication, the results of this trial have been hotly debated, with concerns regarding differences in operator experience between surgeons and interventionalists. Also of note, the stroke rate before the mandatory use of embolic protection devices was extraordinarily high (about 25%) and rates improved significantly after mandatory use of embolic protection devices was put in the study protocol.[16]

Ongoing studies
Several large prospective RCTs are currently enrolling patients. Perhaps the most eagerly awaited study is the Carotid Revascularization Endarterectomy versus Stenting (CREST) trial, which is funded by the National Institutes of Health (NIH). This trial plans to randomize 2500 patients to CEA or CAS and follow-up for 4 years. Optimal current medical management is provided to both arms and intervention is performed in symptomatic patients with 50% stenosis by angiography (70% by ultrasound) and in asymptomatic patients with 60% stenosis by angiography (70% by ultrasound). Some data from this trial has been published indicating an increased risk for octogenarians undergoing CAS.[17] Other ongoing trials comparing CEA and CAS are the International Carotid Stenting Study (ICSS) evaluating low-risk symptomatic patients and the ACT 1 trial, which is evaluating low-risk asymptomatic patients. The Transatlantic Asymptomatic Carotid Intervention Trial (TACIT) will enroll asymptomatic patients to undergo CEA, CAS, or best medical management only. This trial is necessary because the best medical management represented in the landmark surgical trials was not remotely similar to what has been established as best medical management today.[18]

Carotid angioplasty and stenting technique
Our routine procedure for CAS is as follows. The procedure is performed with moderate sedation allowing for continuous neurologic monitoring. Before the procedure, antiplatelet therapy is initiated with aspirin and clopidogrel for at least 5 days and is continued after the procedure. Preprocedural blood pressure control and initiation of statin therapy is also of paramount importance. All patients who have not undergone prior ipsilateral CEA have external pacemaker pads applied before the start of the procedure as a precaution, if extreme bradycardia is encountered and we also ensure that intravenous (IV) atropine is readily available for rapid administration. Access is usually obtained with a common femoral artery puncture and a thoracic angiogram frequently performed. Anticoagulation with heparin is initiated and care taken to maintain an ACT above 250 seconds for the remainder of the procedure. Selective angiography of the nontarget carotid is usually performed to assess potential collateral circulation. Selective angiography of the target vessel is performed in multiple projections to both confirm the diagnosis of significant carotid artery stenosis and to ascertain the best working projection for the planned intervention (**Fig. 2**). Anteroposterior (AP) and lateral angiograms of the head are also performed as a baseline examination. Next, an exchange length wire is manipulated into a branch of the external carotid artery (ECA) and the diagnostic catheter exchanged over the wire for a 6-French 80- to 90-cm guiding sheath. An embolic protection device is then manipulated across the stenosis and the protection device deployed in the internal carotid artery (ICA) distal to the segment to be treated. Predilatation is then performed if needed with a compliant angioplasty balloon. We tend to be more aggressive in predilatation, as we feel this reduces the need for post-stent deployment dilatation by improving the stent approximation to the vessel wall. Next, an appropriately sized carotid stent is deployed

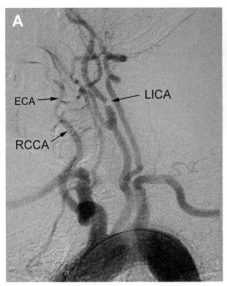
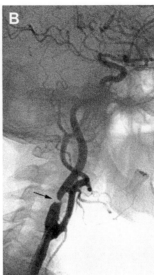
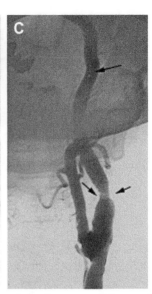

Fig. 2. 57-year-old male with symptomatic left internal carotid artery (ICA) stenosis. (*A*) Left anterior oblique arch arteriogram demonstrates right ICA occlusion and a 98% stenosis of the left ICA approximately 1 cm above the level of the common carotid bifurcation. (*B*) Selective left common carotid artery arteriogram demonstrates 98% eccentric stenosis (*arrow*). (*C*) Poststent arteriogram reveals marked improvement in lumen caliber with mild residual stenosis (*arrow*).

and postdeployment angiography performed. If possible, we avoid poststent deployment balloon angioplasty because it has been our anecdotal experience that a significant number of intraprocedural embolic complications occur during or directly after poststenting balloon angioplasty. This observation may be attributable to a grating effect of the stent on the atheromatous plaque and subsequent emboli during poststenting balloon angioplasty. As a rough guideline, we will accept a 30% or less residual stenosis after stent deployment. Next, the embolic protection device is retrieved and AP and lateral angiograms of the head performed along with a brief on-table neurologic examination. If no complications are encountered, the guiding sheath is exchanged over a wire for a closure device to achieve hemostasis. The patient is then monitored in an ICU setting until the next morning with frequent neurologic examinations and close monitoring of blood pressure.

Long-term efficacy of carotid stenting in terms of stroke prevention appears to be equivalent to carotid endarterectomy but periprocedural morbidity may be increased for patients undergoing carotid stenting. CAS is reserved for selected symptomatic patients with such comorbidities as post CEA re-stenosis, a history of neck irradiation, contralateral laryngeal nerve palsy, anatomically surgically difficult lesions, or poor surgical candidates because of major comorbidities (**Fig. 3**). Low-risk patients should undergo CAS only in the setting of a RCT. Although

currently the standard of care for patients with extracranial carotid stenosis is carotid endarterectomy, it is likely that CAS will have an increasing role to play in the treatment of carotid stenosis in the future. We eagerly await the results of large RCTs comparing the treatment modalities, and to technological improvements to protection devices and stents to further define the role of CAS in the treatment of carotid artery stenosis.

EXTRACRANIAL VERTEBRAL ARTERY STENOSIS

About 25% of all strokes involve the posterior circulation.[19] The association between posterior circulation strokes and vertebral artery stenosis is less well defined than the relationship between anterior circulation stroke and carotid stenosis. The vertebral artery origin is the most common location for vertebral artery stenosis and tends to be associated with adjacent atherosclerosis in the subclavian artery (similar to renal artery stenosis and aortic disease). One registry[20] found 20% of patients with symptoms of vertibrobasilar ischemia to have a proximal vertebral artery stenosis (defined as at least 50% stenosis) and about half of these patients also had contralateral lesions. The risk of stroke after posterior circulation transient ischemic attack has been reported between 25% and 29% during 5- to 6-year follow-up.[21] Despite medical therapy with warfarin or aspirin, these patients have a high recurrence and death rate, reported as 16% to 18%.[22]

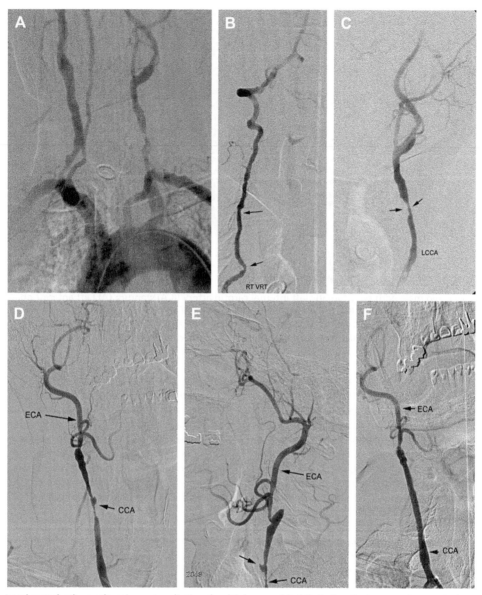

Fig. 3. Accelerated atherosclerosis post radiation (multiple vessels). (*A*) Arch arteriogram demonstrates marked irregularity of both common carotid arteries as well as the origins of the vertebral arteries bilaterally in a patient with laryngeal carcinoma 5 years post radiation therapy. (*B*) Selective right vertebral artery arteriogram demonstrates diffuse irregularity in the proximal vertebral segment. (*B*) Selective left common carotid artery arteriography demonstrates marked irregularity and a focal 1-cm stenosis with ulceration. (*D, E*) AP and lateral views from a right common carotid artery (RCCA) arteriogram in a 63-year-old with history of mantle therapy for lymphoma demonstrates occlusion of the internal carotid artery and a marked stenosis of the common carotid artery with ulceration (*arrow*). The external carotid artery provides collateral flow to the brain via ethmoidal collaterals. (*F*) Following stent placement into the RCCA there was significant improvement in intracranial flow.

A number of case series have been published describing the primary deployment of balloon expandable stents to treat lesions greater than 50% with high technical success rates. These series also report a low incidence of major procedure-related complications (0% to 3.4%) and low incidence of recurrence (1.7% to 3.0%) on short- and intermediate-term follow-up (3 to 37 months). Periprocedural posterior circulation transient ischemic attacks (TIAs) were reported at rates of 0% to 4.8%.[23] Recently, use of an embolic protection device has been advocated during vertebral artery stenting to minimize risk of intraprocedural stroke.[24] The only randomized controlled evaluation of vertebral artery PTA and stenting compared with medical management was a small subgroup of patients within the CAVATAS trial where 16 patients were randomized. Results were nonrevealing owing to the small sample size.[13] A large RCT comparing extracranial vertebral artery stenting with best medical management has yet to be performed. Vertebral artery angioplasty and stenting can be considered as an emerging therapy for patients with symptomatic vertebral artery stenoses that have failed best medical management.

NONATHEROSCLEROTIC ARTERIAL INJURY

Patients with nonatherosclerotic vascular injuries usually present with symptoms, often hemorrhage and/or stroke. This etiologically diverse category encompasses multiple pathologies including trauma (blunt, penetrating, and iatrogenic), vascular injury attributable to cancer or cancer treatment, spontaneous dissection and sequelae, and idiopathic epistaxis. Although these underlying pathologies differ, the diagnostic algorithm and therapeutic approaches are similar allowing us to consider them together.

Management of these patients varies with the acuity of presentation, for example a patient with oral or nasal bleeding, or severe blunt or penetrating trauma, would receive general supportive measures such as airway and hemodynamic resuscitation, before imaging including diagnostic angiogram. CT scan and in many cases CT angiography can be helpful for triage and evaluation of the site of bleeding or vascular compromise. Once the lesion has been diagnosed and defined, diagnostic angiography can be targeted and decisions can be made about appropriate therapeutic options such as distal embolization of the involved vessel, occlusion (sacrifice) of the vessel, or reconstructive endovascular management such as placement of a (covered) stent to treat the lesion. Arteriography must include selective arteriography, assessment of potential collaterals, especially the Circle of Willis, in addition to identification of perilous extracranial-to-intracranial communications that could lead to nontarget embolization if not appreciated.

VASCULAR TRAUMA OF THE FACE AND NECK

Trauma to the extracranial carotid or vertebral arteries may be either blunt or penetrating. Penetrating trauma is by far the more common, with gunshot wounds accounting for most penetrating traumatic injuries in the United States (**Fig. 4**).[25] Although less common, blunt injury to the major arteries of the head and neck can be devastating

with major neurologic morbidity and mortality rates estimated around 60% and 30% respectively.[26] Of all comers to a level 1 trauma center with blunt trauma, 0.24% (37 of 15,331 patients) sustained blunt carotid injury in a study published in 1999. This same study maintained that screening for blunt carotid injury identified a number of asymptomatic patients with serious injuries. Twenty-five of 2902 (0.86%) patients screened were diagnosed with blunt carotid injury and 13 of those (52%) were asymptomatic.[27]

Prompt diagnosis and treatment are critical to patient outcome. CT angiography has become the imaging modality of choice in the emergency room setting. To our knowledge, no comprehensive comparison studies between CTA and angiography exist for screening of trauma patients. CT/CTA findings of vascular injury can vary widely (**Fig. 5**). Frank extravasation of contrast is rarely encountered, but when present, is easily identified as nonvascular contrast. Complete traumatic occlusion of extracranial vessels often involves the cervical ICA 1 to 3 cm above the carotid bifurcation or the vertebral artery at the level of cervical fracture. Intramural hematoma and dissection can result from blunt or penetrating trauma with variable compromise of the involved vessel lumen. Contained rupture of the injured major vessel (pseudoaneurysm) is most often initially irregular in shape but has a tendency to take on a more smooth fusiform or saccular shape over time, depending on the vessel of origin.

Treatment of traumatic injury to the cervical vasculature varies based on the mechanism, type and location of injury, neurologic status, and the presence of associated injuries. Extensive concurrent injuries may preclude the use of antiplatelet regimen needed to place and sustain covered stent graft placement for major vessel injury. With penetrating traumatic vascular injury, diagnostic angiogram followed by endovascular treatment targeted specifically to the injury including distal vessel embolization with particulates, or liquid embolic agents. With blunt traumatic injury leading to pseudoaneurysm or traumatic dissection seen on CTA, without hemorrhage or stroke, treatment decisions are less clear cut. Many advocate close observation in these patients, and if no contraindications exist, treatment is with an anticoagulation/antiplatelet regimen, as complications from these injuries are usually embolic. However, if serial imaging demonstrates interval worsening of imaging findings, or the patient becomes symptomatic from the lesion, intervention may be necessary. Vertebral artery dissection and/or occlusion may be initially treated with vertebral artery sacrifice to prevent recanalization and subsequent

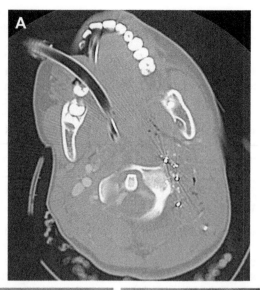

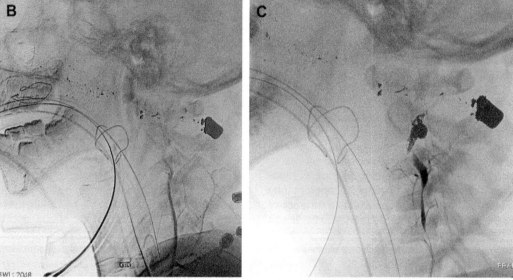

Fig. 4. (*A*) Axial CT following gunshot wound to the right nose demonstrates bullet fragments traversing the course of the vertebral artery at C-1. (*B*) Lateral subtracted arteriogram demonstrates the path and occlusion of the vertebral artery proximal to the metallic fragments. (*C*) The vertebral artery was occluded with platinum coils below the level of the bullet fragments with contrast stasis demonstrated in the distal arterial remnant.

distal embolization and stroke, particularly in patients requiring cervical manipulation or other surgery (**Fig. 6**). A recent review of the literature found favorable results for placement of covered stents in the setting of ICA pseudoaneurysm (**Fig. 7**).[28] If major vessel occlusion is seen on the CTA, endovascular options are limited. Although there have been some good outcomes with opening occluded carotids in the setting of atherosclerotic disease, there are few data on recanalizing traumatically occluded vessels. Emergent surgical bypass and/or thrombectomy are seldom used in this setting.

CAROTID BLOWOUT SYNDROME

Carotid blowout syndrome (CBS) is defined as the rupture of the extracranial carotid arteries or one of its major branches, with oral, nasal, or peritracheal bleeding and has been coined in the setting of head and neck neoplasm, most often squamous cell carcinoma. Carotid blowout is the most feared sequela of head and neck cancer. Prior radiation therapy or brachytherapy are believed to play a key role in the pathogenesis of carotid blowout, possibly because of the obliterating effects on the vasa vasorum caused by radiation and the associated weakening of the arterial wall. Prior

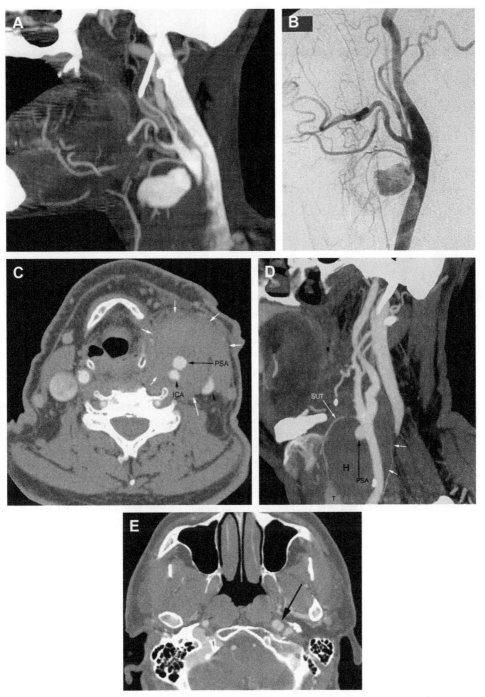

Fig. 5. CTA findings of vascular injury. (*A*) Oblique reformat CTA image demonstrates a pseudoaneurysm originating from the distal common carotid artery at the level of the bulb with an expanding left cervical mass. (*B*) Lateral left common carotid arteriogram demonstrates the opacification of the pseudoaneurysm limit with draping of the superior thyroid artery around partially thrombosed portion of the mass. (*C*) Axial CTA following endarterectomy in a patient with expanding left cervical hematoma, demonstrates pseudoaneurysm at the level of the anastomosis, best illustrated in continuity on the oblique reformatted image (*D*). (*E*) Axial CTA demonstrates typical appearance of a distal cervical ICA dissection with pseudo aneurysmal dilatation.

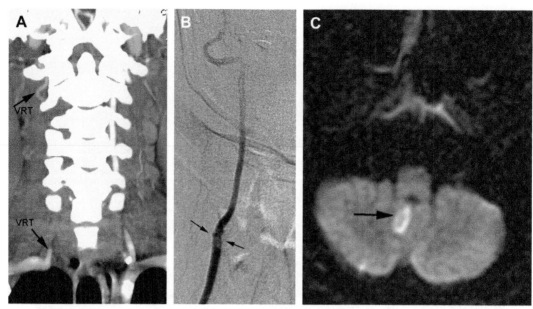

Fig. 6. (A) A 29-year-old male status post motor vehicle accident with bilateral perched facets and apparent vertebral artery (VRT) occlusion. Note the proximal and distal segments of the vertebral artery (*arrows*). (B) Arteriogram 5 days later demonstrates recanalization of the vertebral artery and focal irregularity at the level of the perched facets (*arrows*). (C) MRI diffusion weighted imaging demonstrates restrictive diffusion (*arrow*) consistent with infarct in the distal vertebral territory.

radiation treatment has been associated with a sevenfold increase of CBS in patients with head and neck cancer.[29] Although not confined within the classic definition of carotid blowout syndrome, it is important to keep in mind that significant hemorrhage can also occur from erosion of tumor into the internal jugular vein and from the tumor itself. In the past few years there has been significant improvement in both diagnosis and treatment of CBS.

The reported incidence of CBS in patients with a history of neck dissection is reported to range from 3% to 4%.[30] In the past, carotid blowout has resulted in very significant mortality and morbidity. Recent improvement in care has markedly reduced both mortality and morbidity.[31] Carotid blowout is now approached as a syndrome, with manifestations that can range from acute life-threatening hemorrhage to asymptomatic encasement of a carotid artery. CBS can be categorized into one of three categories: threatened, impending, and acute carotid blowout. Threatened carotid blowout is defined as physical examination or imaging results that suggest inevitable hemorrhage from one of the carotid arteries or its branches if no action is taken. Impending carotid blowout (also called sentinel hemorrhage) is defined as transient hemorrhage that resolves spontaneously or with packing/pressure. Acute carotid blowout represents hemorrhage that cannot be controlled by packing or pressure.[32]

Once carotid blowout syndrome is clinically suspected, the conventional gold standard for diagnosis has been digital subtraction angiography (DSA). However, we believe that noncontrast CT and/or CT angiography have an important role in diagnosis in clinically stable patients. It is useful to understand the extent of tumor, prior surgery, or region treated with brachytherapy seeds before angiography (**Fig. 8**). Unfortunately, there is a lack of literature on the sensitivity and specificity of angiography, and to our knowledge, there is no direct comparison between DSA and CTA for evaluation of carotid blowout syndrome.

Management and Angiographic Approach to Carotid Blowout Syndrome

Initial management of these complex patients revolves around the airway. Controlling the airway is paramount and intubation to prevent aspiration is necessary. Oral, nasal, or wound packing is adjunctive to fluid resuscitation measures and transfusion. Manipulation of the neck wound should be minimized. Once the patient has been stabilized, direct diagnostic and therapeutic strategies can be used.

It is critically important to discuss treatment options and expectations with the patient and/or family representatives with regard to decision making regarding stroke/death risk versus

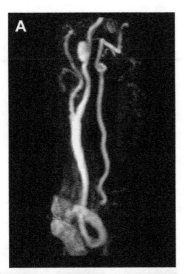

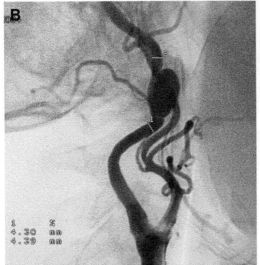

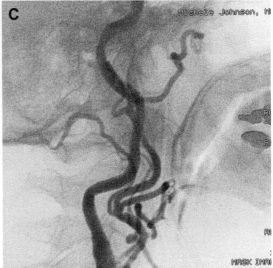

Fig. 7. (*A*) MRA multiple intensity projection (MIP) image in a patient with chronic neck pain demonstrates pseudoaneurysm of the internal carotid artery near the skull base. Following angiographic confirmation (*B*), overlapping stents were placed using a protection device to exclude the pseudoaneurysm from the circulation (*C*).

bleeding/death risk in the treatment of CBS. Patient and family wishes and preferences, including resuscitation status, should be taken into account if bleeding cannot be stopped without significant stroke risk. There are some patients who prefer not to accept the risk of carotid occlusion in spite of the grave prognostic implications of untreated CBS.

Diagnostic angiography varies slightly based on the nature and location of the hemorrhage. Bilateral imaging of the common carotids, the internal carotids, the external carotids, and the vertebral arteries will establish the bleeding site as well as the integrity of the Circle of Willis. This is important in patients who may require carotid artery sacrifice. Selective external carotid branch arteriography is often required to identify a bleeding site

not demonstrable on more global injections.[31,33] Internal maxillary, facial, lingual, ascending pharyngeal, and superior thyroid arteries are the vessels most commonly affected. In patients with peritracheal bleeding, the thyrocervical trunks must also be examined bilaterally.

MAJOR VESSEL LESIONS

During the initial angiographic assessment, catheter placement should be proximal to the suspected carotid injury. The location of surgical clips and brachytherapy seeds are local indicators of the potential site of vascular compromise. For frank rupture, sacrifice of the carotid artery above and below the point of rupture will prevent the

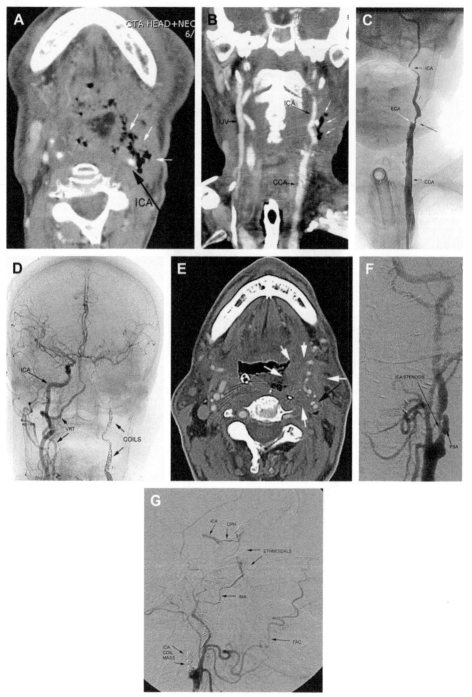

Fig. 8. (*A–D*) A 72-year-old status post salvage laryngectomy for squamous cell carcinoma of larynx with intractable oral bleeding. Axial (*A*) and coronal (*B*) CTA demonstrates air (*white arrows*) dissecting within the carotid space directly adjacent to the left internal carotid artery (ICA) (*black arrow*) and a local soft tissue mass. Note the absence of the internal jugular vein (IJV) on the left. (*C*) AP LCCA arteriogram demonstrates marked irregularity of the distal CCA, stenosis at the origin of the ICA with marked irregularity to the level of the skull base. A stump (*white arrow*) is seen at the origin of the external carotid artery. (*D*) AP RCCA angiogram demonstrates robust collaterals filling the left intracranial vasculature from the right ICA and the right vertebral arteries. Note the coil mass on the left. (*E–G*) A 60-year-old male with nasopharyngeal carcinoma and oral bleeding. (*E*) Narrowing of the internal carotid artery with a small angular contrast collection consistent with pseudoaneurysm within a soft tissue tumor mass (*white arrows*). The IJV is occluded. (*F*) Angiography confirms the PSA and the adjacent ICA stenosis. (*G*) The ICA and the PSA were permanently occluded using detachable platinum coils. Control arteriography demonstrates prompt filling of distal ethmoidal branches of the IMA to collateralize with the ophthalmic artery (OPH) that is filling retrogradely to reconstitute the supraclinoid ICA.

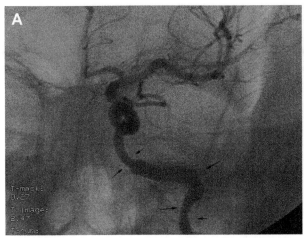 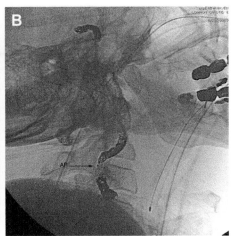

Fig. 9. A62-year-old patient 2 weeks post endoscopic resection of presumed recurrent nasopharyngeal carcinoma. (*A*) AP view of a left internal carotid artery (ICA) arteriogram demonstrates narrowing and irregularity of the petrous internal carotid artery (*arrows*) adjacent to the site of recent surgery. (*B*) Following successful left ICA BOT, the ICA was occluded permanently using a combination of platinum detachable coils and the Amplatzer Plug (AP).

creation of a pattern of unreachable collateral flow. Often both the internal and external carotid branches must be occluded (see **Fig. 8**). Carotid sacrifice was formerly performed with detachable silicone or latex balloons; however, these are not currently available in the United States. Currently we perform carotid sacrifice with detachable coils, with variable adjunctive use of the Amplatzer vascular plug (AGA Medical Corporation, Plymouth, MN) for occlusion of the proximal aspect of the vessel (**Fig. 9**).

In CBS patients with a lesion of the common or internal carotid, such as pseudoaneurysm, ulceration, or long-segment irregularity, sacrifice of the involved carotid may be the only life-saving option. Ideally, when time permits, a temporary balloon occlusion test (BOT) is performed to ascertain tolerance of carotid artery occlusion before the procedure. The three components of a temporary balloon occlusion test include diagnostic arteriography for collateral assessment, clinical testing during temporary occlusion, and TC-hexamethyl-propyleneamine oxime–single-photon emission computed tomography (HMPAO-SPECT) or xenon CT evaluation of cerebral blood flow during temporary occlusion. Balloon occlusion testing is further described elsewhere in this issue.

Covered stent (stent graft) placement has been used for salvage of major vessels in carotid blowout. This technology is limited in the setting of open wounds, active infection, and unfavorable anatomy. The use of covered stents may be an option in some patients; however, one must be prepared to convert a stent procedure into carotid occlusion if hemostasis cannot be maintained

(**Fig. 10**).[34,35] When carotid sacrifice cannot be safely performed because of lack of collateral flow or a lack of tolerance of temporary balloon occlusion testing, and stent placement is not an option, surgical extracranial-to-intracranial bypass techniques may be considered, in association with carotid sacrifice, to augment cerebral blood flow.[36]

When CBS manifests as uncontrollable hemorrhage, carotid sacrifice must then be performed without clinical preocclusion testing (as a life-saving procedure). In this situation, HMPAO-SPECT is sometimes performed following occlusion to assist in postocclusion ICU hypertensive and hypervolemic management. The occlusion balloon is withdrawn and the carotid sacrificed using retrievable and/or detachable coils. Alternatively, the occlusion balloon catheter can be left in place with the balloon inflated and a microcatheter advanced through the lumen of the occlusion balloon and embolization of the distal ICA performed during balloon occlusion of the proximal ICA. This allows immediate control of bleeding and the ability to raise blood pressure to enhance cerebral perfusion during the permanent occlusion. Clinical management in the ICU includes neurologic monitoring and hemodynamic measures to maintain cerebral perfusion pressure. CT scan of the head can be adjunctive following patient stabilization.

NON–MAJOR VESSEL SOURCES OF HEMORRHAGE

Significant oral, nasal, or peritracheal bleeding may result from tumoral neovascularity or erosion

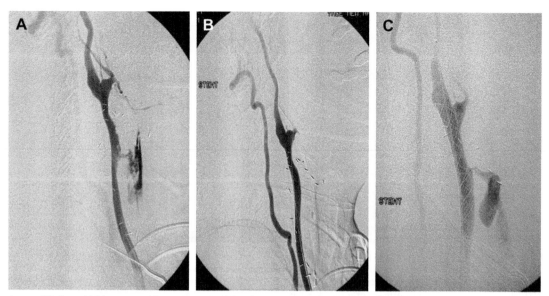

Fig. 10. (*A*) Carotid blowout with massive oral bleeding into the pharynx demonstrates marked irregularity with extravasation. Note extensive radiation seeds. (*B*) Following failed BOT, two overlapping covered stents were placed in the common carotid artery with the achievement of hemostasis. (*C*) Twenty-four hours later, there was recurrent oral bleeding, and despite placement of two additional overlapping stents, contrast extravasation was again demonstrated. The carotid artery was sacrificed permanently. The patient survived without neurologic deficit for 18 months. (*From* Johnson MH. Carotid blowout syndromes. Endovascular Today 15–18 Jan/Feb 2003; with permission.)

through the wall of a small external carotid branch vessel, rather than major vessel erosion. Selective external carotid branch arteriography is often required to demonstrate the bleeding site. Microcatheterization both permits identification of the bleeding site and allows for more selective placement of embolic material. Selection of embolic material depends on the site and the nature of the hemorrhage source. In our experience, in the trauma setting, embolization is most often performed with particulate such as polyvinyl alcohol foam (PVA) or gelfoam, with or without adjunctive placement of coils. In the setting of head and neck cancer, radiation, and infection, liquid embolic agents are more durable in these fragile, diffusely diseased vessels (**Fig. 11**).

TUMORAL HEMORRHAGE

Hemorrhage derived from neovascularity of the tumor or local granulation tissue can be treated with medium-sized, 250-micron to 350-micron particles of PVA suspended in dilute contrast media. We introduce the particles into the tumor under roadmap guidance using a microcatheter and 1-cc syringes until the neovascularity is sufficiently reduced. Proximal gelfoam pledgets may be adjunctive. This is a temporizing measure that may allow for healing of friable tumor. One should

avoid using small 50-micron to 150-micron particles if additional surgery is not planned, to avoid frank tumor necrosis and subsequent secondary infection.

VASCULAR LACERATION OR PSEUDOANEURYSM

Vascular laceration or pseudoaneurysm (PSA) may be treated directly with microcatheter embolization to address the specific bleeding site in the setting of trauma or head and neck cancer/tumor/radiation (CBS). Embolic materials vary with the setting. Gelfoam with or without complex helical coils may be used for a discrete vessel laceration in the setting of trauma. This will control bleeding in an otherwise intrinsically normal lacerated vessel; we use Trufill n-BCA Liquid Embolic System (Cordis Corporation, a Johnson & Johnson company, Miami, FL), where possible, for pseudoaneurysm or focal extravasation (**Fig. 12**). Proximal vessel coil embolization should be avoided, because it does not directly address the site of pathology. In most cases, when attempts at proximal occlusion have failed to control hemorrhage, small microcatheters can navigate beyond proximally placed clips or coils for more distal embolization. When choosing an embolic agent, pay attention to the site of the lesion, the nature of adjacent collaterals, the distal

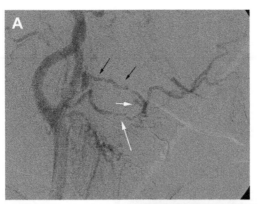

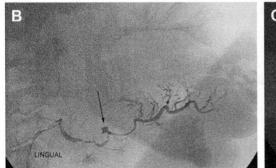

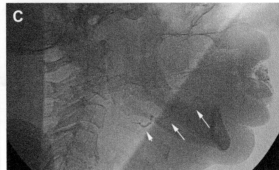

Fig. 11. (A) Lateral common carotid artery angiogram in a patient with a base of tongue cancer demonstrates marked irregularity of the facial artery (*black arrow*) and marked narrowing and irregularity with pseudoaneurysm of the lingual artery. (B) Selective lingual arteriogram demonstrates marked narrowing and irregularity and a pseudoaneurysm of the lingual artery at the tongue base. (C) The lingual artery and pseudoaneurysm were embolized with NBCA (see the radio-opaque glue cast in the lingual artery after embolization).

parenchymal territory, and the role of embolization (ie, presurgical or palliative).

EXTRACRANIAL CAROTID AND VERTEBRAL ARTERY SPONTANEOUS DISSECTION

Arterial dissection is an intimal tear in the wall of an artery allowing intrusion of blood products within the layers of the arterial wall. As this hematoma in the false lumen between the intima and media expands, it may compress the true lumen, resulting in stenosis, occlusion, and/or pseudoaneurysm formation with weakening of the media and adventitia. Spontaneous or nontraumatic dissection of the extracranial carotid and vertebral dissection were once thought to be rare, but may account for as many as 20% of strokes in patients younger than 45 years.[37]

The pathogenesis of spontaneous dissection is incompletely understood. A history of minor neck trauma is often present although not universal. Patients with underlying connective tissue disorders such as fibromuscular dysplasia, Ehlers-Danlos syndrome, Marfan's syndrome, and alfa 1 antitrypsin deficiency syndrome may be more vulnerable to cervical vascular dissection. There has been speculation that recent infection may play a role in the pathogenesis of dissection, in part supported by some seasonal variance.[38] It has also been speculated that migraine history, hypertension, and smoking may contribute to increased risk of dissection.

Carotid and vertebral dissection are classified into extradural (extracranial) and intradural (intracranial) dissections. Extradural/extracranial dissection is far more common although intradural extension of dissection is usually more significant and carries a poorer prognosis and a risk of subarachnoid hemorrhage. Spontaneous dissection is more common in the carotid arteries (80%) than in the vertebral arteries.[39] The arterial segments affected differ between dissection and atherosclerosis. Dissection often involves the distal part of the ICA near the point of fixation at the entry into the carotid canal at the skull base, whereas atherosclerosis most often affects the carotid bulb and the origin of the ICA. Vertebral dissection frequently occurs near points of fixation such as the entry or exit from the foramen transversarium and where the vertebral artery pierces the dura at the

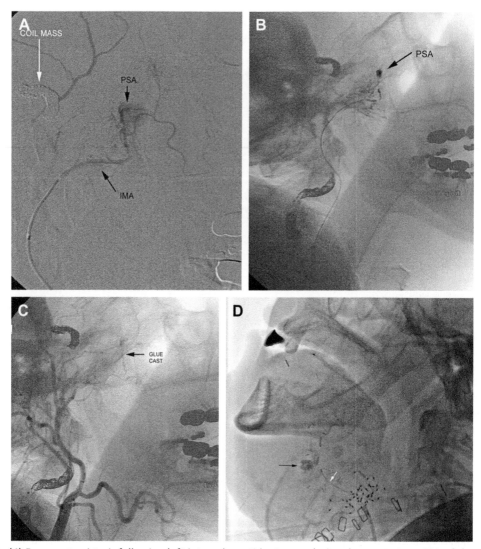

Fig. 12. (*A*) Recurrent epistaxis following left internal carotid artery occlusion demonstrates a PSA of the second portion of the IMA. (*B*) Acrylic glue is identified within the PSA. (*C*) Oral bleeding 7 days post resection and graft placement for treatment of floor of mouth cancer demonstrates a PSA of the graft at the anastomosis (*white arrows*). (*D*) Acrylic glue cast demonstrated within the PSA. The graft remained viable.

foramen magnum. Atherosclerosis tends to involve the origin of the vertebral artery.

Classic clinical features of spontaneous dissection are often not present, but include neck pain, Horner's syndrome, headache, cranial nerve palsies, and neurologic deficits secondary to distal embolization or ischemia from flow compromise. Embolic phenomena are most common because of platelet aggregation at the site of injury and distal embolization. A study from 2004 demonstrated territorial infarcts (presumed embolic in origin) in all patients with dissection contrasted with watershed infarcts (secondary to hemodynamic phenomena) in only 5% of these patients.[40]

Extracranial dissection is readily diagnosed with noninvasive methods such as Doppler ultrasound, MRI/MR angiography (MRA), and most recently with CT angiography (CTA). Identification of the false lumen filled with thrombus on the T1 fat saturation image is diagnostic. Irregularity of the lumen or sharp edges rather than curves on the axial CTA images are equally diagnostic when the studies are technically of good quality (**Fig. 13**). Catheter angiography is usually performed only for problematic cases or when intervention is considered.

Treatment is essentially medical and rarely do these patients require endovascular or operative management. Once diagnosed, thromboembolism is the most feared possible sequalae. Management

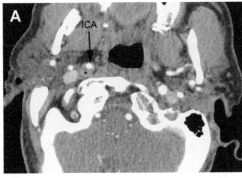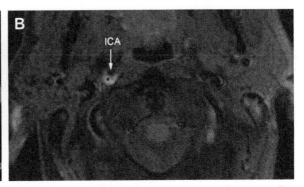

Fig. 13. (A) Axial CTA demonstrates a spontaneous dissection of the internal carotid artery with surrounding thrombus (*). Spontaneous dissection is similarly well demonstrated on fat-saturation T1-weighted images (B).

revolves around minimizing the risk of embolic phenomenon using antiplatelet agents as the mainstay of treatment. In cases with severe luminal compromise, short-term heparin and/or warfarin administration is sometimes used.

The prognosis depends largely on the severity of neurologic deficit incurred before diagnosis, but is generally good with vessel wall healing with extracranial dissection. Recurrence rates are very low in the absence of underlying connective tissue disease.

IDIOPATHIC EPISTAXIS

A majority of the adult population will experience epistaxis during their lifetime although only a small minority will experience bleeding requiring medical attention.[41] There is a small group of patients who do not respond to conservative therapies such as local packing. Epistaxsis is deemed idiopathic if there is no known underlying etiology such as trauma or tumor. These patients are treated with various forms of therapy including posterior and anterior packing, vasoconstrictors, endoscopic cautery, surgical ligation and/or endovascular embolization. Patients with posterior epistaxis are said to be particularly difficult to manage conservatively and often require a more aggressive treatment regimen including endovascular embolization.[42] Endovascular embolization of idiopathic epistaxis was first described in 1974 by Sokoloff and colleagues.[43] Since that time, numerous series have been published detailing results and technique. A recent review of the literature showed an average technical success rate of 88% and average postprocedural complication rate to be 12%.[44] The most common agent used in these series was PVA, with particle size varying from 50 to 750 micrometers although many different distal particulates were used such as embospheres and gelfoam. Endovascular embolization

has a high success rate and low morbidity rate. Primary success rates range from 79% to 96% with recurrence after embolization ranging from 0% to 24%. Major complications secondary to epistaxis embolization were rare, 3%, consisting of stroke (most common), monocular blindness, skin sloughing, ICA dissection and postprocedural MI.[44] Minor complications such as self-limiting facial pain and numbness have also been described. Randomized comparison of embolization to other forms of treatment, such as surgery, have not been performed.

An important caveat is worth mentioning. Epistaxis in the setting of hereditary hemorrhagic telangiectasia (HHT or Osler-Weber-Rendu disease) is, in our experience, refractory to effective treatment with embolization. It has been our experience and confirmed in the literature that patients with HHT do not have a durable result after embolization and fare much better with operative septal dermoplasty as the initial therapeutic strategy to control severe epistaxis.[45]

When performing endovascular embolization for epistaxis, a complete diagnostic angiogram is absolutely essential. This includes detailed evaluation of the external and internal carotid arteries. The primary vascular supply to the nasal mucosa includes the internal maxillary and distal facial arteries (**Fig. 14**). The distal most branches of the ophthalmic artery may also contribute and may become more prominent following embolization of the internal maxillary and facial nasal supply. Rarely, epistaxis may be caused by internal carotid pathology, particularly in the setting of prior radiation treatment or trauma (see **Fig. 9**). Evaluation of the ICA is also critical to minimize the risk of nontarget embolization and to delineate anastamoses between the ECA and ICA circulations. It has been our experience that a definite bleeding site is very infrequently seen during angiography for idiopathic epistaxis. Traditionally,

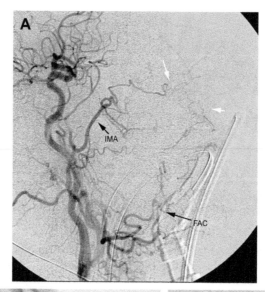

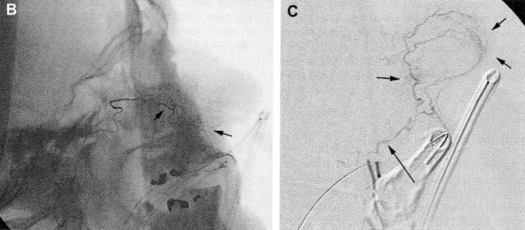

Fig. 14. (*A*) The blood supply to the nasal mucosa and septum is derived from the IMA and facial artery (FAC), which provide a balanced circulation (*white arrows*). (*B*) Microcatheter injection into the distal internal maxillary nasal branches demonstrates a normal nasal arterial arcade. (*C*) Distal facial microcatheter arteriogram demonstrates extensive arterial vascular supply to the nasal mucosa and septum.

embolization for idiopathic epistaxis has involved angiography of the distal nasal branches of the internal maxillary and facial arteries followed by particulate (PVA) embolization of three of the four branches (usually both distal internal maxillary artery [IMA] and the dominant facial artery) to reduce the opportunity for collateral flow to friable nasal vessels before they have time to heal. A key component to decision making is laterality. If the side of bleeding has been determined before angiography, some authors feel that single-vessel embolization, usually the IMA is sufficient for control. The ipsilateral facial nasal branches may then be embolized if there is significant vascular contribution to the nasal mucosa.[46]

SUMMARY

It is imperative for the neuroendovascular specialist to be proficient with diagnosis and treatment of common extracranial pathologies. For atherosclerotic vascular disease, technologies continue to improve and potentially expand the role of endovascular techniques for treatment while study trials are ongoing and results are anxiously awaited to determine the ultimate role of CAS in disease management. For traumatic vascular injury, embolization for vessel closure and vessel preservation using stents and stent grafts are a routine part of patient management. Although carotid blowout remains a challenge for rapid triage and treatment, our expanding tools and aggressive ICU management help many patients to survive potentially catastrophic hemorrhage. The neuroendovascular techniques are uniquely suited to treat a wide variety of extracranial vascular diseases.

REFERENCES

1. Meyers PM, Schumacher HC, Higashida RT, et al. Use of stents to treat extracranial cerebrovascular disease. Annu Rev Med 2006;57:437–54.

2. North American Symptomatic Carotid Endarterectomy Trial Collaborators. Beneficial effect of carotid endarterectomy in symptomatic patients with high-grade carotid stenosis. N Engl J Med 1991;325:445–53.

3. Randomised trial of endarterectomy for recently symptomatic carotid stenosis: final results of the MRC European Carotid Surgery Trial (ECST). Lancet 1998;351:1379–87.

4. Eliasziw M, Smith RF, Singh N, et al. Further comments on the measurement of carotid stenosis from angiograms. North American Symptomatic Carotid Endarterectomy Trial (NASCET) Group. Stroke 1994;25(12):2445–9.

5. Barnett HJ, Taylor DW, Eliasziw M, et al. Benefit of carotid endarterectomy in patients with symptomatic moderate or severe stenosis. North American Symptomatic Carotid Endarterectomy Trial Collaborators. N Engl J Med 1998;339:1415–25.

6. Endarterectomy for asymptomatic carotid artery stenosis. Executive Committee for the Asymptomatic Carotid Atherosclerosis Study. JAMA 1995;273:1421–8.

7. Asymptomatic Carotid Surgery Trial (ACST) Collaborative Group. Prevention of disabling and fatal strokes by successful carotid endarterectomy in patients without recent neurological symptoms: randomized controlled trial. Lancet 2004;363(9420):1491–502.

8. Mayberg MR, Wilson SE, Yatsu F, et al. Carotid endarterectomy and prevention of cerebral ischemia in symptomatic carotid stenosis. Veterans Affairs Cooperative Studies Program 309 Trialist Group. JAMA 1991;266:3289–94.

9. Results of a randomized controlled trial of carotid endarterectomy for asymptomatic carotid stenosis. Mayo Asymptomatic Carotid Endarterectomy Study Group. Mayo Clin Proc 1992;67:513–8.

10. Moore WS, Barnett HJ, Beebe HG, et al. Guidelines for carotid endarterectomy. A multidisciplinary consensus statement from the Ad Hoc Committee, American Heart Association. Stroke 1995;26:188–201.

11. Bockenheimer SA, Mathias K. Percutaneous transluminal angioplasty in arteriosclerotic internal carotid artery stenosis. AJNR Am J Neuroradiol 1983;4:791–2.

12. Naylor AR, Bolia A, Abbott RJ, et al. Randomized study of carotid angioplasty and stenting versus carotid endarterectomy: a stopped trial. J Vasc Surg 1998;28:326–34.

13. Endovascular versus surgical treatment in patients with carotid stenosis in the Carotid and Vertebral Artery Transluminal Angioplasty Study (CAVATAS): a randomised trial. Lancet 2001;357:1729–37.

14. Yadav JS, Wholey MH, Kuntz RE, et al. Protected carotid-artery stenting versus endarterectomy in high-risk patients. N Engl J Med 2004;351:1493–501.

15. Ringleb PA, Allenberg J, Bruckmann H, et al. 30 day results from the SPACE trial of stent-protected angioplasty versus carotid endarterectomy in symptomatic patients: a randomised non-inferiority trial. Lancet 2006;368:1239–47.

16. Mas JL, Chatellier G, Beyssen B, et al. Endarterectomy versus stenting in patients with symptomatic severe carotid stenosis. N Engl J Med 2006;355:1660–71.

17. Hobson RW, Howard VJ, Roubin GS, et al. Carotid artery stenting is associated with increased complications in octogenarians: 30-day stroke and death rates in the CREST lead-in phase. J Vasc Surg 2004;40:1106–11.

18. Gaines PA, Randall MS. Carotid artery stenting for patients with asymptomatic carotid disease (and news on TACIT). Eur J Vasc Endovasc Surg 2005;30:461–3.

19. Bogousslavsky J, van Melle G, Regli F. The Lausanne Stroke Registry: analysis of 1,000 consecutive patients with first stroke. Stroke 1988;19:1083–92.

20. Wityk RJ, Chang HM, Rosengart A, et al. Proximal extracranial vertebral artery disease in the New England Medical Center Posterior Circulation Registry. Arch Neurol 1998;55:470–8.

21. Hornig CR, Lammers C, Butter T, et al. Long term prognosis of intratentorial transient ischemic attacks and minor strokes. Stroke 1992;23:199–240.

22. Mohr JP, Thompson JL, Lazar RM, et al. A comparison of warfarin and aspirin for the prevention of recurrent ischemic stroke. N Engl J Med 2001;345:1444–51.

23. Zavala-Alarcon E, Emmans L, Little R, et al. Percutaneous intervention for posterior fossa ischemia. A single center experience and review of the literature. Int J Cardiol 2008;127:70–7.

24. Henry M, Polydorou A, Henry I, et al. Angioplasty and stenting of extracranial vertebral artery stenosis. Int Angiol 2005;24:311–24.

25. Davis JM, Zimmerman RA. Injury of the carotid and vertebral arteries. Neuroradiology 1983;25:55–69.

26. Cogbill TH, Moore EE, Meissner M, et al. The spectrum of blunt injury to the carotid artery: a multicenter perspective. J Trauma 1994;37:473–9.

27. Biffl WL, Moore EE, Ryu RK, et al. The unrecognized epidemic of blunt carotid artery injuries. Ann Surg 1999;228(4):462–9.

28. Maras D, Lioupis C, Magoufis G, et al. Covered stent-graft treatment of traumatic internal carotid artery pseudoaneurysms: a review. Cardiovasc Intervent Radiol 2006;29:958–68.

29. Maran AGD, Amin M, Wilson J. A radical neck dissection: a 19 year experience. J Laryngol Otol 1989;10:760–4.

30. Koch WM. Complications of surgery of the neck. In: Eisele D, editor. Complications in head and neck surgery. St Louis (MO): Mosby; 1993. p. 393–413.

31. Morrissey DD, Andersen PE, Nesbit GM, et al. Endovascular management of hemorrhage in patients with head and neck cancer. Arch Otolaryngol Head Neck Surg 1997;123(1):15–9.

32. Chaloupka JC, Roth TC, Putman CM, et al. Recurrent carotid blowout syndrome: diagnostic and therapeutic challenges in newly recognized subgroup of patients. AJNR Am J Neuroradiol 1999;5:1069–77.

33. Chaloupka JC, Putman CM, Citardi MJ, et al. Endovascular therapy for the carotid blowout syndrome in head and neck surgical patients: diagnostic and managerial considerations. Am J Neuroradiol 1996; 17:843–52.

34. Lee S, Huddle D, Awad IA. Indications and management strategies in therapeutic carotid occlusion. Neurosurg Q 2000;10:211–23.

35. Roth TC, Chaloupka JC, Putman CM, et al. Percutaneous direct-puncture acrylic embolization of a pseudoaneurysm after failed carotid stenting for the treatment of acute carotid blowout. Am J Neuroradiol 1998;19(5):912–6.

36. Toyoda T, Sawatari K, Yamada T, et al. Endovascular therapeutic occlusion following bilateral carotid artery bypass for radiation-induced carotid artery blowout: a case report. Radiat Med 2000;18(5): 315–7.

37. Bogousslavsky J, Pierre P. Ischaemic stroke in patients under age 45. Neurol Clin 1992;10:113–24.

38. Grau AJ, Brandt T, Buggle F, et al. Association of cervical artery dissection with recent infection. Arch Neurol 1999;56:851–6.

39. Schievink WI, Mokri B, Whisnant JP. Internal carotid artery dissection in a community: Rochester, Minnesota, 1987–1992. Stroke 1993;24:1678–80.

40. Benninger DH, Georgiadia D, Kremer C. Mechanism of ischaemic infarction in spontaneous carotid dissection. Stroke 2004;35:482–5.

41. Shaw CB, Wax MK, Wetmore SJ. Epistaxis: a comparison of treatment. Otolaryngol Head Neck Surg 1993;109:60–5.

42. Sinuloto TM, Leinonen ASS, Karttunen AI, et al. Embolization for the treatment of posterior epistaxis. Arch Otolaryngol Head Neck Surg 1993;119:837–41.

43. Sokoloff J, Wickborn I, McDonald D, et al. Therapeutic percutaneous embolization in intractable epistaxis. Radiology 1974;111(2):285–7.

44. Christensen NP, Smith DS, Barnwell SL, et al. Arterial embolization in the management of posterior epistaxis. Otolaryngol Head Neck Surg 2005;133: 748–53.

45. Layton KF, Kallmes DF, Gray LA, et al. Endovascular treatment of epistaxis in patients with hereditary hemorrhagic telangiectasia. AJNR Am J Neuroradiol 2007;28:885–8.

46. Johnson MH, Chiang VL, Ross DA. Interventional neuroradiology adjuncts and alternatives in patients with head and neck vascular lesions. Neurosurg Clin N Am 2005;16:547–60.

Index

Note: Page numbers of article titles are in **boldface** type.

A

Abciximab, for stroke, 420
ACAS (Asymptomatic Carotid Atherosclerosis Study),
 488
ACST (Asymptomatic Carotid Surgery Trial), 488
Alcohol, for embolization
 of dural arteriovenous malformations, 438
 of intracranial arteriovenous malformation
  embolization, 411–412
Alligator retrieval device, for stroke, 425
Alteplase, for stroke, 420, 422
Anesthesia
 for aneurysm treatment, 384
 for arteriovenous malformation treatment,
  407–408
Aneurysm(s)
 intracranial
  arteriovenous malformations with, 405–406
  asymptomatic, 383
  endovascular treatment of, **383–398**
   anesthesia for, 384
   angiography in, 394
   balloon-assisted coiling technique,
    391–393
   clinical trial outcomes of, 387–390
   complications of, 394–395
   deconstructive approach to, 393
   follow-up in, 394
   Guglielmi detachable coil system, 390–391
   indications for, 383
   Jefferson Hospital experience with,
    385–387
   Onyx HD 500, 393
   patient selection for, 384–386
   postoperative care in, 393–394
   reconstructive approach to, 390–393
   stent-assisted coiling technique, 391
   technical aspect of, 384–385
  risk factors for, 383
  rupture of, intraprocedural, 394–395
 "intranidal," 403
 subarachnoid hemorrhage after, endovascular
  treatment of, **441–446**
Aneurysmal venous ectasia, in dural arteriovenous
 malformations, 433
Angiography
 in carotid blowout syndrome, 496
 in carotid cavernous fistulas, 448–450
 in carotid trauma, 493

in craniocervical tumor embolization, 475
in dural arteriovenous malformations, 465
in intracranial aneurysms, 394
in intracranial arteriovenous malformations,
 402–403
in stroke, 420
AngioJet system, for stroke, 425
Angioplasty
 balloon, for vasospasm, after subarachnoid
  hemorrhage, 442–444
 carotid, 488–491
Antegrade perfusion, for stroke, 425
Anticoagulation, for aneurysm treatment, 384
Arteriovenous malformations
 dural, **431–439, 463–474**
  anatomic considerations in, 432–436
  classification of, 431–432
  clinical features of, 432–436
  endovascular treatment of, 436–438
   convexity type, 469, 471–474
   palliative embolization in, 466–467
  imaging of, 436
 intracranial, **399–418,** 453–463
  aneurysms with, 405–406
  clinical presentation of, 400
  diagnosis of, 402–403
  endovascular treatment of, 402–412
   anesthesia for, 407–408
   case examples of, 461–463
   classification of, 454
   complications of, 412–413, 460
   curative embolization in, 406
   embolic agents for, 408–412
   embolization technique for, 454–459
   goals of, 399
   indications for, 453–454
   large/giant type, 456–457
   outcomes of, 461
   palliative embolization in, 406–407
   postprocedural care in, 413, 459–460
   preoperative embolization in, 404
   preradiosurgery embolization in, 404–405
   procedure for, 407–408
   targeted embolization in, 405–406
   with fistulas, 460–461
  epidemiology of, 399–400
  grading of, 401–402
  mortality in, 401–402
  natural history of, 400–401
  pathogenesis of, 400

doi:10.1016/S1042-3680(09)00104-1

neurosurgery.theclinics.com

United States Postal Service

Statement of Ownership, Management, and Circulation
(All Periodicals Publications Except Requestor Publications)

1. Publication Title	2. Publication Number								3. Filing Date
Neurosurgery Clinics of North America	0	1	3	—	1	2	1	4	9/15/09

4. Issue Frequency	5. Number of Issues Published Annually	6. Annual Subscription Price
Jan, Apr, Jul, Oct	4	$274.00

7. Complete Mailing Address of Known Office of Publication (Not printer) (Street, city, county, state, and ZIP+4®)

Elsevier Inc.
360 Park Avenue South
New York, NY 10010-1710

Contact Person
Stephen Bushing

Telephone (Include area code)
215-239-3688

8. Complete Mailing Address of Headquarters or General Business Office of Publisher (Not printer)

Elsevier Inc. 360 Park Avenue South, New York, NY 10010-1710

9. Full Names and Complete Mailing Addresses of Publisher, Editor, and Managing Editor (Do not leave blank)

Publisher (Name and complete mailing address)

John Schrefer, Elsevier, Inc., 1600 John F. Kennedy Blvd. Suite 1800, Philadelphia, PA 19103-2899

Editor (Name and complete mailing address)

Ruth Malwitz, Elsevier, Inc., 1600 John F. Kennedy Blvd. Suite 1800, Philadelphia, PA 19103-2899

Managing Editor (Name and complete mailing address)

Catherine Bewick, Elsevier, Inc., 1600 John F. Kennedy Blvd. Suite 1800, Philadelphia, PA 19103-2899

10. Owner (Do not leave blank. If the publication is owned by a corporation, give the name and address of the corporation immediately followed by the names and addresses of all stockholders owning or holding 1 percent or more of the total amount of stock. If not owned by a corporation, give the names and addresses of the individual owners. If owned by a partnership or other unincorporated firm, give its name and address as well as those of each individual owner. If the publication is published by a nonprofit organization, give its name and address.)

Full Name	Complete Mailing Address
Wholly owned subsidiary of	4520 East-West Highway
Reed/Elsevier, US holdings	Bethesda, MD 20814

11. Known Bondholders, Mortgagees, and Other Security Holders Owning or Holding 1 Percent or More of Total Amount of Bonds, Mortgages, or Other Securities. If none, check box → ☐ None

Full Name	Complete Mailing Address
N/A	

12. Tax Status (For completion by nonprofit organizations authorized to mail at nonprofit rates) (Check one)
The purpose, function, and nonprofit status of this organization and the exempt status for federal income tax purposes:
☐ Has Not Changed During Preceding 12 Months
☐ Has Changed During Preceding 12 Months (Publisher must submit explanation of change with this statement)

PS Form 3526, September 2007 (Page 1 of 3 (Instructions Page 3)) PSN 7530-01-000-9931 PRIVACY NOTICE: See our Privacy policy in www.usps.com

---

13. Publication Title		14. Issue Date for Circulation Data Below
Neurosurgery Clinics of North America		April 2009

15. Extent and Nature of Circulation		Average No. Copies Each Issue During Preceding 12 Months	No. Copies of Single Issue Published Nearest to Filing Date
a. Total Number of Copies (Net press run)		1332	1127
b. Paid Circulation (By Mail and Outside the Mail)	(1) Mailed Outside-County Paid Subscriptions Stated on PS Form 3541. (Include paid distribution above nominal rate, advertiser's proof copies, and exchange copies)	484	459
	(2) Mailed In-County Paid Subscriptions Stated on PS Form 3541 (Include paid distribution above nominal rate, advertiser's proof copies, and exchange copies)		
	(3) Paid Distribution Outside the Mails Including Sales Through Dealers and Carriers, Street Vendors, Counter Sales, and Other Paid Distribution Outside USPS®	281	270
	(4) Paid Distribution by Other Classes Mailed Through the USPS (e.g. First-Class Mail®)		
c. Total Paid Distribution (Sum of 15b (1), (2), (3), and (4))	→	765	729
d. Free or Nominal Rate Distribution (By Mail and Outside the Mail)	(1) Free or Nominal Rate Outside-County Copies Included on PS Form 3541	66	41
	(2) Free or Nominal Rate In-County Copies Included on PS Form 3541		
	(3) Free or Nominal Rate Copies Mailed at Other Classes Through the USPS (e.g. First-Class Mail)		
	(4) Free or Nominal Rate Distribution Outside the Mail (Carriers or other means)		
e. Total Free or Nominal Rate Distribution (Sum of 15d (1), (2), (3) and (4))	→	66	41
f. Total Distribution (Sum of 15c and 15e)	→	831	770
g. Copies not Distributed (See instructions to publishers #4 (page 83))	→	501	357
h. Total (Sum of 15f and g)	→	1332	1127
i. Percent Paid (15c divided by 15f times 100)	→	92.06%	94.68%

16. Publication of Statement of Ownership

☐ If the publication is a general publication, publication of this statement is required. Will be printed in the October 2009 issue of this publication. ☐ Publication not required

17. Signature and Title of Editor, Publisher, Business Manager, or Owner

Stephen R. Bushing

Stephen R. Bushing – Subscription Services Coordinator

Date September 15, 2009

I certify that all information furnished on this form is true and complete. I understand that anyone who furnishes false or misleading information on this form or who omits material or information requested on the form may be subject to criminal sanctions (including fines and imprisonment) and/or civil sanctions (including civil penalties).

PS Form 3526, September 2007 (Page 2 of 3)

Moving?

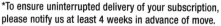

Printed and bound by CPI Group (UK) Ltd, Croydon, CR0 4YY

03/10/2024

01040360-0011